A YEAR WITH

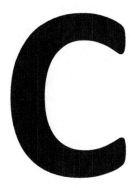

CANCER, CREATIVTY, CLAIRE

BY CLAIRE JAMES

Author's Biography

Claire is an artist, primary school teacher and became an author after being diagnosed with Breast cancer. She used creativity to share her journey through treatment. She was born in West Sussex and has lived most of her life in the South East. In her spare time, she enjoys being in the outdoors and going for long walks with the family and her dog, Moose.

For Milo, my anchor in the storm.

Acknowledgment

First and foremost, I would like to thank my mum, who not only came up with this idea but has been my rock over the last year, for my whole life in fact. You are the most selfless, caring person I know and I simply could not do it without you.

Thank you to Harry - my husband, best friend and life partner who took care of me & Milo, in spite of his own pain, I am so grateful for your positivity and strength. You make the good days amazing and the bad days bearable.

To my family; my dad and brothers Dan & Dunc, for the cuddles and LOLs when I needed them most. To my sister KEB for being my number one cheerleader. To my in laws, Ian, Sarah, Tom and Tara for being there for me and Harry and helping with Milo when I wasn't able. Thank you to all my extended family, near and far, for providing lots of love & laughter and helping me make some wonderful memories during this turbulent year.

Thank you to my friends; Ella for dropping everything to come and take care of me after chemo, Meg for not only being a wonderful friend but also being my personal nurse at times,

Rose for all the love and delicious food, the college girls for monthly care packages, Rory and Ish for being such brilliant friends as well as my creative advisors and finally, all the others for sending heartfelt messages, thoughtful gifts and beautiful flowers, which kept me going on my lowest days. I will never forget your kindness.

Thank you to the NHS and the staff at the Royal Surrey Hospital for saving my life, in particular Nana, Sam and Claire and the other nurses of the Teenagers and Young Adults Cancer ward, for taking such good care of me.

Lastly, thank you to Michelle and my team at the Book Writing Founders for helping to put this book together and bringing my vision to life.

Foreword by Rory Langdon-Down

Creativity takes courage - Henri Matisse.

365 days is a really, really long time. I expect that not many of you have ever counted every single day in a year as it passes, feeling the weeks move by at a pace of somehow both the tortoise and the hare. Claire has.

When I heard about Claire's cancer diagnosis at the end of 2021, I asked if she was going to document her new unknown world in any way. She answered without hesitation. The fact that her creativity would play a vital role in her journey was one of very few certainties she had at the time, so with a tidal wave approaching and little idea what was behind it, Claire gripped to what she knew - her family, her friends, and a blank sketchbook.

That first sketchbook became what you're looking at today. 365 days of creativity that documents every part of Claire's story throughout 2022. This book is both a piece of art in its own right and a tangible guide that reveals the intricacies of cancer. Where words can't convey what pictures can, Claire has created an insight not only into her life with cancer, but the beautiful day-to-day aspects of life that will feel familiar to all of us.

When you dedicate yourself to a project of this magnitude, there are no hiding places. No hiding from creative self-doubt (an unfortunate pre-requisite of an artist); no hiding from the rawness of cancer and the physical and emotional effects on you and your family; and no hiding from the mundaneness of a typical

day when everything is actually just sort of 'fine'. Days of 'nothing to report'. Those are the days that make you question the point of creating anything at all - but that's the point. The days we all take

for granted are the ones Claire longed for, and the unredacted inclusion of all of these moments are what gives this project its power.

A Year with C harnesses the courage Claire used to beat cancer. However, these pages also represent the invaluable help that her work provides friends, family and strangers. Creating art with that kind of significance is rare and for years to come this book will continue to share the courage it stores.

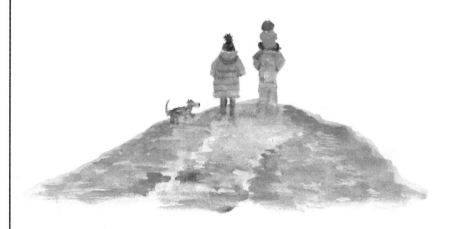

CONTEMPLATING THE YEAR AHEAD.

I have been debating whether to do this for a while. After being diagnosed with breast cancer at 31 years old, I have been on an emotional rollercoaster, torn between whether to go inside myself or share my experience with others. So, I have decided to go with the latter, with some good advice and kind motivation that it is completely under my control. Now, if anything, I'm excited to see where this will lead me.

CLOUDY WITH BURSTS OF SUNSHINE.

Today was a grey and wet day, but we did manage to get out for a muddy walk. In the afternoon, my family came round for dinner, which was lovely as always. The next time I see them, I'll probably have a shaved head and, hopefully, some cool tattoos.

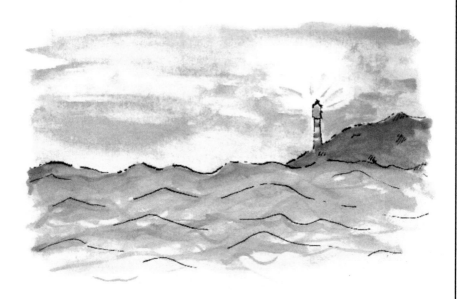

STORMY SEAS AHEAD.

The thought of the year ahead fills me with dread and makes my stomach do back flips. However, I know that I am stronger than the storm, especially with the amazing support system I have in my family and friends. The little one, in particular, will be my anchor in the storm.

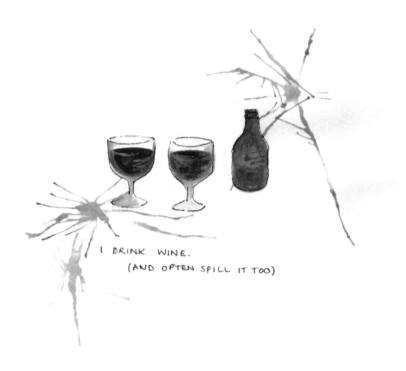

I DRINK WINE.
(AND OFTEN SPILL IT TOO)

... far too often at the moment. The nice thing is Harry finally likes wine now, so we can enjoy a bottle together. This is also a nod to my favourite song and Adele's new album, which happened to come out around the time of my diagnosis, so it has become a real medicine for both of us.

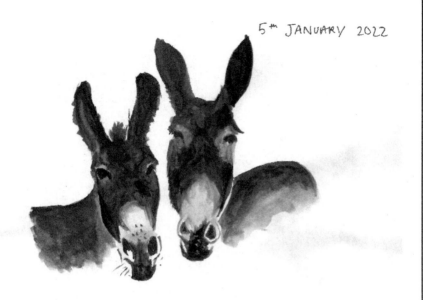

IOW DONKEY SANCTUARY.

Today we took the little man to see the donkeys. As we pulled into the car park, I got a call from the nurse in the X-ray department, booking me into another biopsy tomorrow. It made the visit feel slightly strange and reminded me how this disease will constantly weave into my life from now on. We had a great time visiting the donkeys, and I even got a nice cosy hat to keep my hairless head warm.

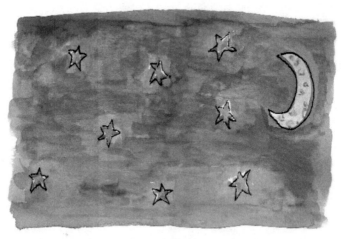

FRIENDS ARE LIKE MOON & STARS IN THE DARKNESS.

Telling family and friends has been the hardest thing about cancer. However, I have been floored by the love and support I have received, and I count myself incredibly lucky to have such a wonderful, caring and thoughtful support system.

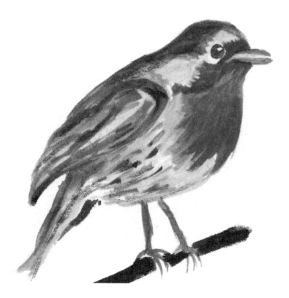

SITTING, WATCHING, WAITING.

One of my favourite things about our new house is sitting and watching all the birds in our garden. In particular, I love the robins as they remind me of my aunt, who we lost in August. I will probably spend a lot of time in this spot on the sofa over the next year, so I feel so lucky to be able to watch the birds and the garden as it changes through the seasons.

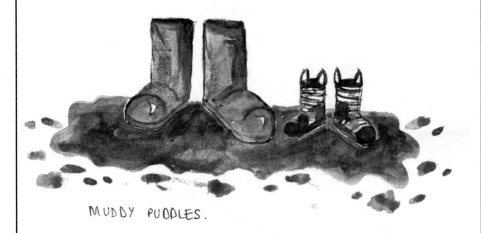

MUDDY PUDDLES.

Sheesh! Today was wet and miserable. Pathetic fallacy, you might say. It was a quiet day, which was nice after such a busy time recently. We did manage to get out for a walk this afternoon but got drenched on the way back. The little one really is my favourite person to go tramping with, and I love that he has a growing interest in nature.

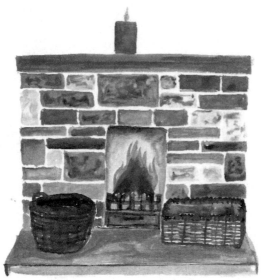

COSY NIGHTS IN.

On cold days like today, my favourite thing is to get a fire going and snuggle up with my team. I feel in a state of limbo at the moment, waiting for my treatment to start. Constantly reviewing how I might feel/react to the chemo is quite frankly exhausting. Luckily, my family keeps me distracted, and it was nice of them to join me in getting creative this evening.

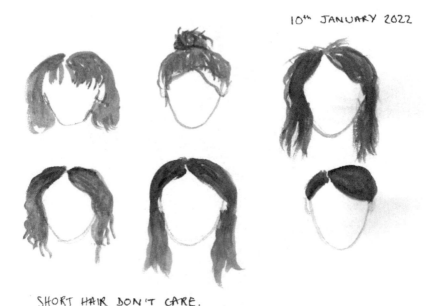

SHORT HAIR DON'T CARE.

My relationship with my hair has always been love-hate. I have been blessed with thick hair from the day I was born but have struggled to tame it most of my life. I have tried a fair few styles over the years to try and combat it, some of which I have loved, some I have done myself and some which went straight into a messy bun on top of my head. But life has a funny way of throwing things at you, and now that I'm being presented with losing my hair entirely, I regret ever cursing it. Anyway, worst things have happened, and I was spoilt rotten today having my hair cut short, so it's not so much of a shock when it falls out. Biggest thank you to my best pal Meg for booking it, sitting by my side throughout, and being a total babe.

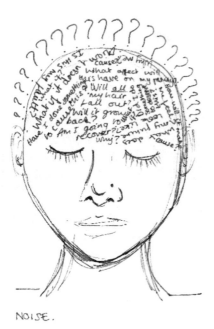

NOISE.

Today was a quiet day which means my head is a cacophony of questions, some of which I don't dare ask out loud. Most don't have answers.

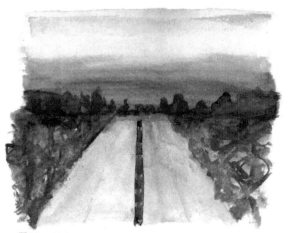

THE ROAD.

I have recently spent a lot of time driving up and down the motorway for various hospital appointments. I actually love being alone in my car as I can have whatever music I like rather than 'Room on the broom' for the thousandth time, and it's my favourite thinking time. The sky was phenomenal tonight, and after a long meeting with the chemo nurse, I need to focus on the 'hope & light' at the end of the tunnel.

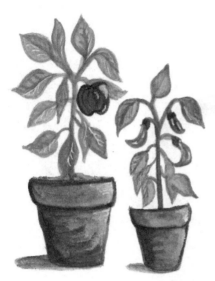

PATIENCE.

We were given these pepper plants when we first moved into our house last summer, and I put them in the green house to start growing. The little peppers began to appear in autumn, so I brought them inside for warmth. The large pepper started green but is slowly changing colour. I can't actually bring myself to pick them, as I want to see if it will eventually turn red. It's a waiting game. Much like the year ahead of me, it's all about patience and trusting the process.

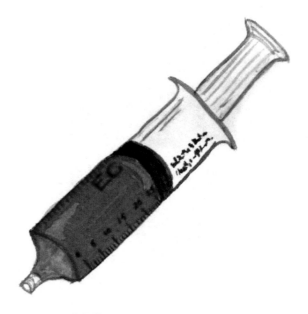

THE FIRST DOSE.

Today I started chemo, which was a surreal experience. You see those wards on tv and never actually imagine yourself sitting in one. The type I am having has to be administered by a nurse with a syringe, so she sat with us the whole time and was so lovely. We were laughing and joking throughout, which made it much easier. It's a strange feeling being injected with something that will make you sick to kill the thing that isn't making you feel sick? Bizarre. It's the start of a long journey and the first of many visits to the chemo ward, but I'm on the way to getting better.

YUCK.

Today was a rough day. Felt sick (hence the colour) and spent most of the day on the sofa. I hate not being able to play with my little one or even get out for a walk, but I guess this is all part of the journey. Thank god for my amazing team, my incredible husband, my wonderful mother and my beautiful friends for keeping me fed and giving me lots of cuddles.

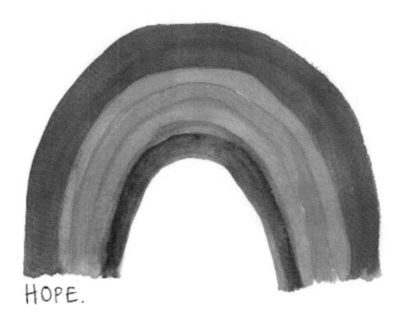

HOPE.

Today was a better day. Managed to keep down food and actually get out for a short walk in the sunshine. This gives me a huge amount of hope that not every day will be as bad as yesterday. Hopefully, I will continue to feel better tomorrow and then be able to have some good days before the next dose.

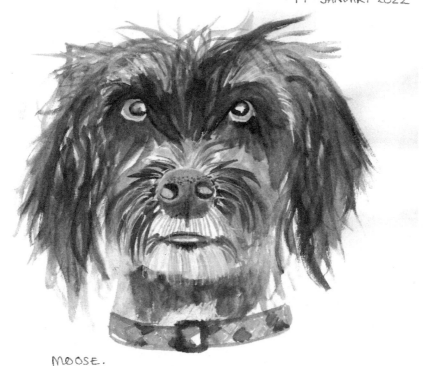

MOOSE.

Today was another slow day slumped on the sofa at Mum's. Moose barely left my side today as if she could sense I needed some comfort. At one point she even lay across my tummy like a hot water bottle. My little fur baby.

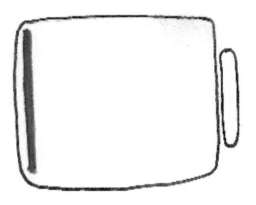

BATTERY LOW.

Tired, wiped, drained. It's hard to stay positive on days like today, but I've got my little cheerleaders around me. We can do this.

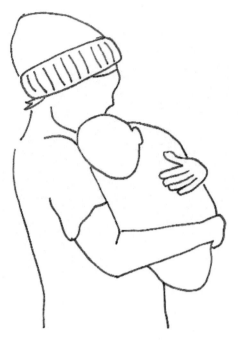

MOTHERHOOD.

Today I got my first cuddles with a close friend's baby, which made my heart full. It took me back to the early days with my little boy and made me crave those slow days of feeding and sleeping. The impact of this disease on my son is the thing that worries me the most. I can't be the Mum I want to be to him at the moment, but I know that he will understand, and the times I have been curled up on the sofa, he comes to sit with me and says, "I'm here, Mummy." Luckily, he has an incredible Daddy who is looking after us both.

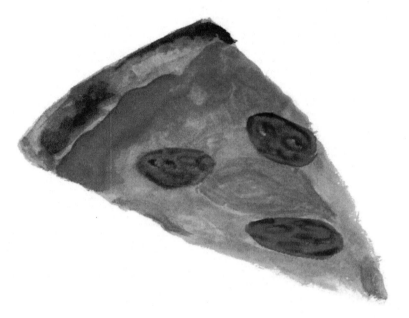

FUEL.

I love food. Always had a huge appetite, even when I wasn't feeling great until last week. After my first dose of chemo, the sickness meant I had no interest in food whatsoever, and it's taken a while to come back. Harry has just popped out to get us a pizza which I'm looking forward to and hoping we will be able to enjoy!

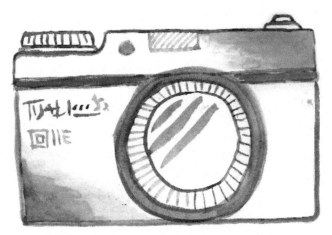

CAPTURING THE GOOD TIMES.

Today we had a visit from our wonderful friend Rory who is Milo's Godfather and also an incredible photographer who has captured some amazing memories over the years.

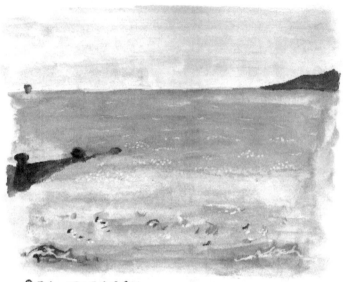

SEA THERAPY.

I took a walk along the beach today, followed by a (very) quick
dip with my Mum - Something we're trying to do more often
after being constantly told about the health benefits and
seeing a good friend totally addicted. I've always loved being
by the sea, more so in winter as I just find it so calming and
therapeutic.

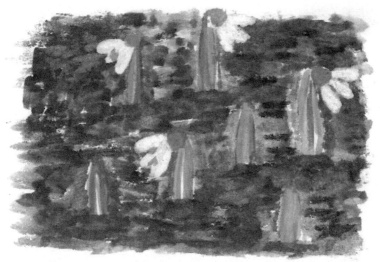

SIGNS OF SPRING.

The snowdrops are starting to creep up through the soil in my garden, which is a welcome surprise and makes me feel like spring is on its way. It's nice to imagine the garden in full bloom again and being able to sit outside in the sunshine.

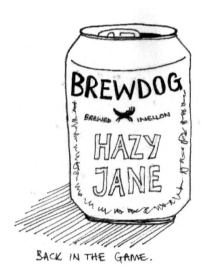

BACK IN THE GAME.

Feeling sick is a little like a hangover and puts you off from having any kind of alcohol. So when I actually felt like a beer this evening, it was a relief! The thought of getting through this year without alcohol felt a little drab, so being able to enjoy a drink in between treatments is great.

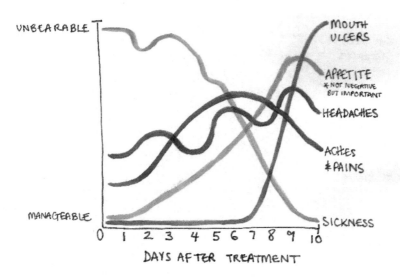

SYMPTOMS.

In honour of my talented best friend, Ella, I have used infographics this evening to portray the array of symptoms I've experienced and their severity. Honestly, the splashes of colours make an ugly thing quite pretty!

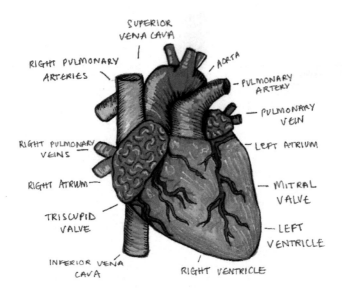

THE HEART.

Today I had a PICC line put in which I can have my chemo put through and blood taken from. In order to find my vein, he used ultrasound and showed me the difference between the artery and the vein, which reminded me of GCSE biology learning about the heart. I always found it fascinating, as well as infuriating trying to remember all the parts. I also found out today that I have to start taking 2 types of medication to protect my ticker from the chemo.

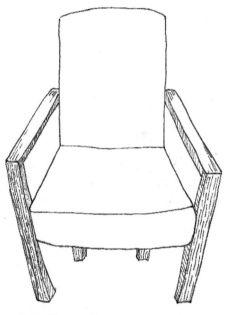

ROUND TWO.

The second dose of EC today, on the TYAC ward which was so lovely, and the nurses were amazing. I was absolutely dreading it, and as the sickness creeps in this evening, it is hard knowing what's to come. But equally, I know that normality will return, I just gotta get my head down and push on through. Thank you to all my wonderful friends and family for the support.

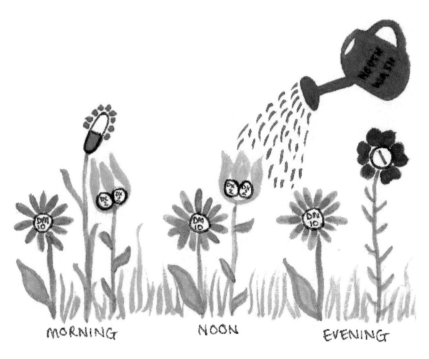

MORNING   NOON   EVENING

A DAY OF MEDICATION.

Trying to make my medication look pretty. This is now what I
have to take in a day to counter the effects of the chemo;
Domperidone - anti-sickness Ramipril - heart medication x2
anti-sickness with steroids. Ondansetron - anti sickness
Mouthwash for the ulcers. +paracetamol for headaches and
Gaviscon for acid reflux from taking all these pills. I actually
feel lucky that I'll only be on this many for a short while. Some
people have to take this many pills every day of their life. Also
so thankful I have an amazing medical team and have access
to this treatment in the first place!

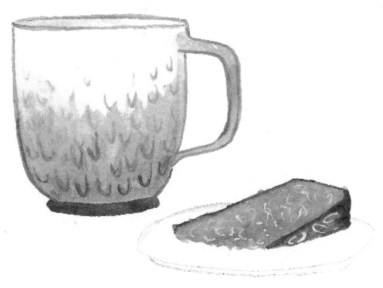

TEA AND CAKE.

Today was a quiet day spent on the sofa at my parents' house as Harry was away for the weekend. Mum has been looking after me all day and keeping me fed and watered, including this delicious orange & almond cake. Thanks Mama; you're amazing.

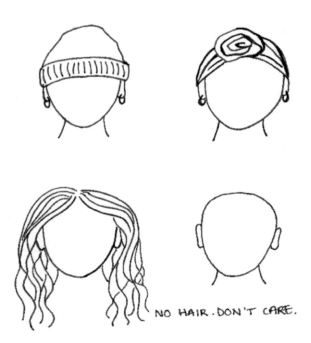

NO HAIR · DON'T CARE.

My hair is starting to come out. I can run my hand through and pull it out easily. It's funny; I thought it wouldn't bother me. There's so much else going on in my body that I thought it would be the least of my worries. But I feel sad, probably because my hormones are askew, and that now I really am going to 'look' as sick as I feel. I know it's going to come back, and I know it's a tiny part of who I am, but it still feels strange. It was the first thing people used to say about me "look at all that hair." Luckily, I already had a few headpieces ready to go, including a nice wig, and have prepped Milo that I am going to look like a baby, which he finds funny.

38

THERE IS A WAR GOING ON
INSIDE MY BODY,

THE CANCER IS THE FEARED,
YET IT IS THE CHEMO
THAT IS MAKING ME SICK.

THERE IS A WAR GOING ON
INSIDE MY BODY.

BUT I CAN'T HELP THINKING,
WHAT IS GOING TO BE LEFT?

Didn't have the energy to paint today, but this poem came
into my head when I couldn't sleep last night.

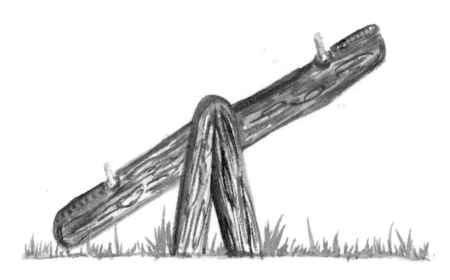

SEESAW.

Took Milo to the park with Mum today, and all 3 of us went on the seesaw, which was actually a lot of fun until we started feeling dizzy. I feel like this is how my mind is at the moment, constantly flipping between "this f*cking sucks" and "god, I'm so lucky; it could be so much worse." It's exhausting, but thankfully, most of the time, I land on the latter.

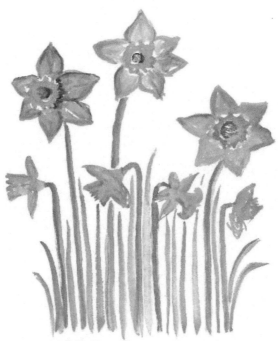

WARMER DAYS.

The weather was beautiful today, and it felt warm while we were out in the garden. We even spotted this group of daffodils that were a bit early to the party but a welcome sight that made me look forward to warmer days.

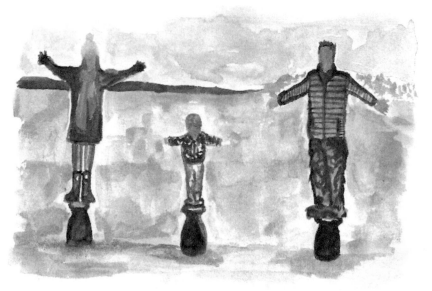

BABA'S BIRTHDAY.

It was my Dad's birthday, so we went down to the beach. It was a pretty gloomy day, but the colours were amazing, and we spent most of the time watching Milo throw stones into the sea, chased by Moose. I made them line up for this shot for old times' sake as we used to do it all the time as kids.

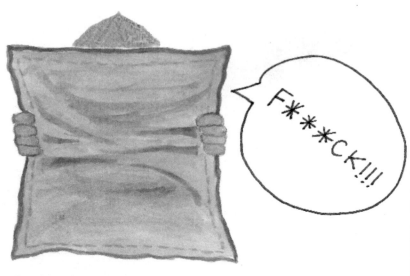

FUCK YOU CANCER.

Today was a hard day. I was up with Milo most of last night then he was acting up all morning and testing me. I wanted to scream at him, though I knew it's not his fault. It's just another reminder of this horrible disease, and its impact on my loved ones. Luckily, my amazing family was there to help and scoop him up so I could sleep. On days like today, all I really feel like saying is Fuck You Cancer.

5th FEBRUARY 2022

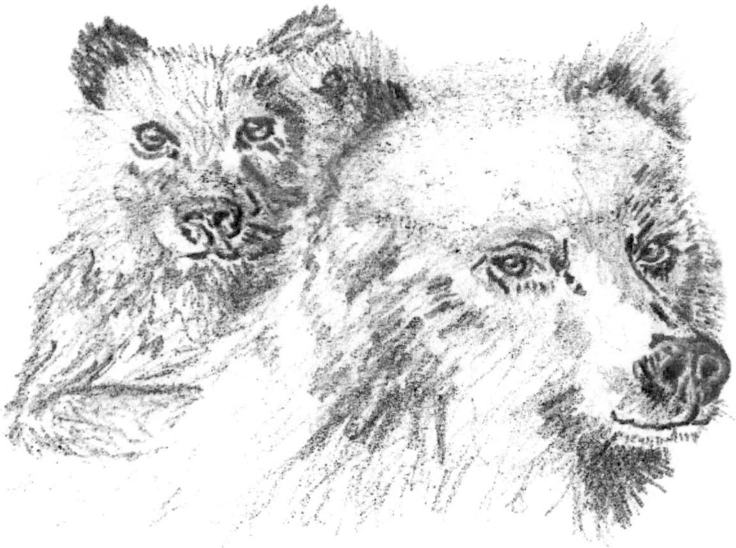

MAMA BEAR.

What a difference a day makes. Milo slept much better last night, which meant we all did, so I woke up feeling like a human again. We went for a play in the park and then to a great garden centre with my family, and everyone was in good form. It makes a world of difference. Motherhood is a rollercoaster of emotions, and your mood often depends on theirs, so I try to make sure days like these are treasured the most.

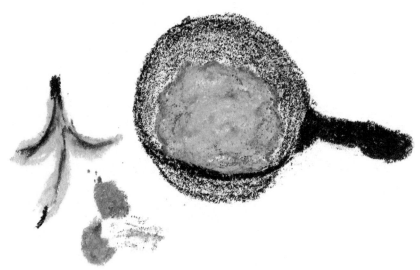

BANANA PANCAKES.

This morning was my favourite kind. Milo had a lie in, then woke up in a great mood, and we had an easy start to Sunday by making banana pancakes together. Then my wonderful friend Lottie popped by with lovely gifts, including some oil pastels, which I had a go with this evening. Finally, my family came over for an early tea which rounded off the weekend. Feeing very thankful tonight and lucky to have such loving friends and family.

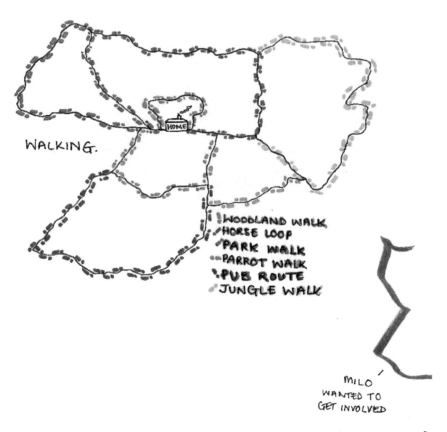

WALKING.

WOODLAND WALK
HORSE LOOP
PARK WALK
PARROT WALK
PUB ROUTE
JUNGLE WALK

MILO
WANTED TO
GET INVOLVED

One of the best things about our new house is the amount of
walks we have on our doorstep. On the days I feel rubbish, I
can barely get off the sofa, so on days like today when I have
energy, I love being able to get out. Milo was at nursery this
morning, so it was just me and moose in the sunshine.

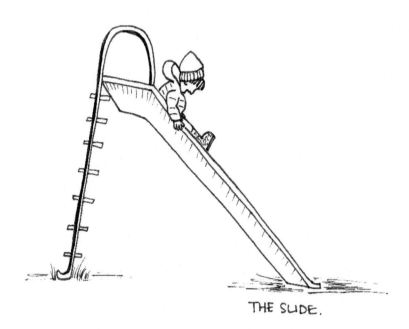

THE SLIDE.

Back to the park with Milo today, he spent about 20 minutes going up and down the slide without the pleasure seeming to fade. It's quite a good metaphor for how I feel after treatment; it's a steep climb out of fatigue and sickness, then when I reach the top and feel like myself again, I begin the slide back down, which goes all too quickly. As I approach my 3rd round, I feel the anxiety build about going through it all over again but got to keep my head up and know it will all be over soon.

47

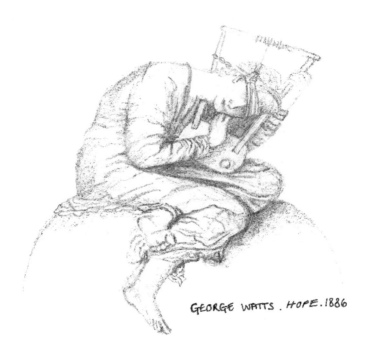

GEORGE WATTS . HOPE. 1886

Today Mum and I visited the Watts Gallery and saw this incredible painting, 'Hope' by George Watts. Supposedly, it inspired Barack Obama to pursue the presidency, and Nelson Mandela had a copy in his prison cell. Standing in front of it, you can see why. The blindfolded figure sitting upon a globe represents humanity, who clings to the lyre straining to hear the music coming from the last remaining string. It's haunting, yet it shows that even in dark times, we will still endeavour to find joy.

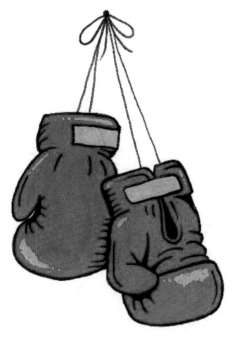

ROUND 3.

Today was my third and final dose of the dreaded 'Red Devil' EC. Knowing what to expect makes it easier, and the wonderful nurses on the ward and being joined by my old pal Ella made the whole experience quite lovely. However, a little bit like a really good night out; the aftermath is no fun at all, but as I know, I will make it out the other side.

Today's picture was inspired by a Simpsons video. My brother sent me Homer in a boxing ring, being hit repeatedly without any effect so that his opponent eventually passes out from exhaustion. I can do this.

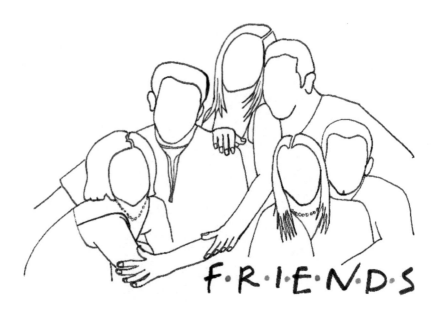

Ella spent the day with me on the sofa, and we watched our favourite show, which we've been watching together for over 20 years now. It's such a classic and is a total comfort blanket. This is also a homage to my incredible friends who have completely blown me away with love and support through this whole thing. From a simple heart on treatment days to parcels filled with chocolate and other treats, I feel so ridiculously lucky. You are all amazing, and I will never forget your kindness and generosity.

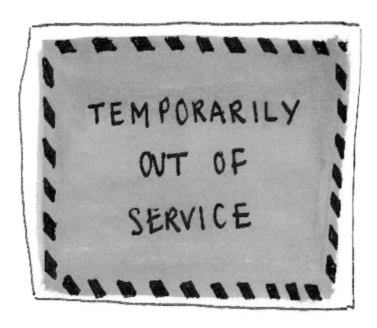

WIPED.

Felt shattered today, and the sickness is trying to rear its ugly head. Doesn't help that this time I had my injection, which suppresses my ovaries, essentially giving me menopause, so I can add that to the list of symptoms. Bleurgh. Anyway, enough moaning. It's another day done and another step closer to the end.

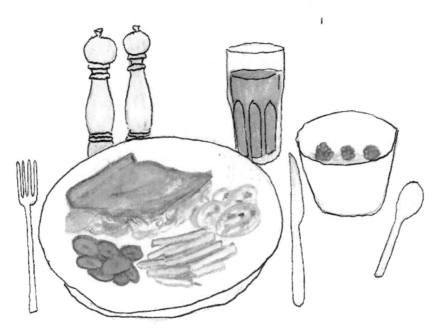

SUNDAY DINNER.

Last night was a horrible night of sickness and hot flushes but made better this morning by a visit from the lovely Emma. Then my brother and girlfriend came over to play board games as the weather was so pants. (Game: Carcassonne 10/10 would recommend) To top it off, Mama arrived with dinner of tasty chicken pie and delicious veg finished off with steamed apple and raspberries. A perfect way to end a rainy Sunday.

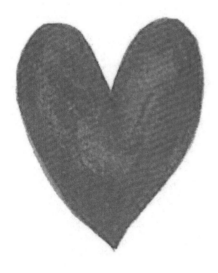

LOVE.

Harry and I have never celebrated Valentine's, but I feel I should use this day to thank him for how incredible he has been through all of this. I can't even begin to imagine how hard this is for him, yet he's being so brave and caring. Love you beyond words

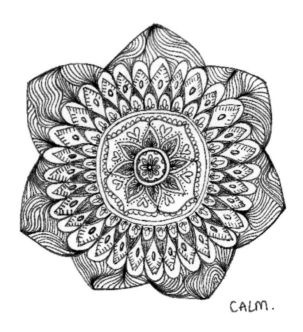

CALM.

Tonight I feel angry. Angry that I'm having to put my body through relentless hell as well as putting my loved ones through so much pain. Angry that I have so little control over what is happening and feel so completely stuck. Maybe I'm just exhausted, maybe it's the menopause irritability, but tonight I'm pissed off. So I drew a Mandela, the process always makes me feel calm, and I genuinely feel better after finishing it. I know there are so many positives, and there is no doubt I will beat this, so chin up, I'm pushing on.

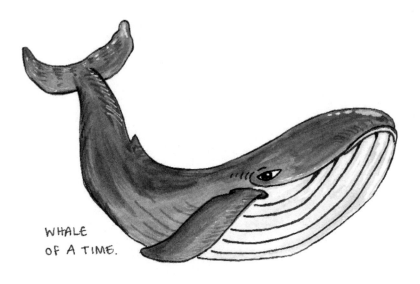

WHALE
OF A TIME.

Milo wanted to read one of our faves today, "Snail and the whale," which I love for its illustrations of far-off lands. It's nice to imagine being able to take him exploring further afield one day and show him this crazy, beautiful world we live in. For now, I'll have to rely on my dreams and cherished memories of better times.

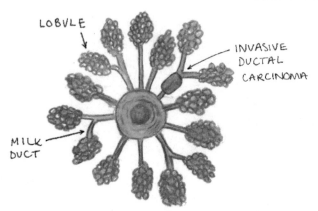

LOBULE

INVASIVE
DUCTAL
CARCINOMA

MILK
DUCT

BREAST CANCER.

I was diagnosed with invasive ductal carcinoma in November 2021. After finding a lump in my right breast and seeing my GP, I was referred for an ultrasound, where they also took a biopsy of the lump, which confirmed it was cancerous and can spread to other areas of the breast tissue. My (very) basic understanding of the science is that cells in the milk ducts start to mutate, then they 'invade' out and cause the lump. It goes without saying that; ladies, check ya breasts, but at the same time, sometimes things don't go as you expect. The treatment plan the doctors have set out for me is rigorous but extremely well-researched, and I trust in them entirely. This journal is a way for me to process what's happening as well as keep family and friends updated, and an added bonus has been connecting with others in the cancer community.

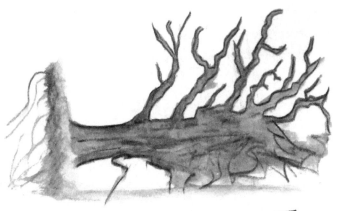

STORM EUNICE.

STORM EU-NOT-NICE.

Now that I feel more human again, we had a lovely morning at soft play with friends, then rushed home to shelter form the storm. The drive was only 5 mins but was pretty hairy, with branches falling all over the road. On arriving home, we realised we had no power, along with half the country, I imagine. The afternoon was spent inside, watching the storm swirl around us. Something comforting in that.

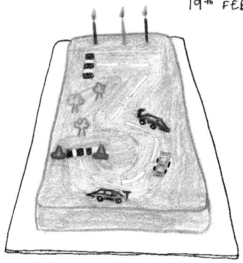

WILBO'S BIRTHDAY PARTY.

Today we travelled to Gloucester for my nephew's 3rd birthday party. It was your absolutely classic, with a bouncy castle in the village hall with balloons, cocktail sausages, and party bags. I spent most of my time on the bouncy castle bopping the balloons at the kids as they collapsed in hysterics. My favourite part was watching the group of 3-year-olds spend 25 minutes trying to smash a piñata until an adult took over as they lost interest. It's such a treasure to be able to enjoy days like these, and I have a new lease of appreciation for the simple pleasures of life.

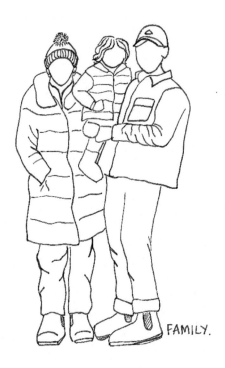

FAMILY.

Tonight I feel grateful. Not only do I have an amazing group of friends and family supporting me through this, but most importantly, have my little team. They make the bad days bearable and the good days amazing. Not everyone going through this will have that, so I feel incredibly lucky. Hopefully, I can make it up to them one day.

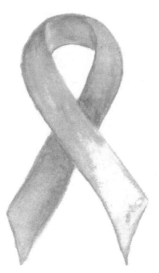

THE CANCER COMMUNITY.

It's not a community you ever think you're going to be part of, but now I am, I have to say I have been absolutely blown away by the support and camaraderie from the people I have met on this journey. Total strangers, with whom the thing we have in common, is so ugly and destructive, have sent me messages of love and encouragement because they know how it feels. Just want to say a huge thank you and send my thoughts and love to all of those who are fighting this horrible disease. You are all superheroes.

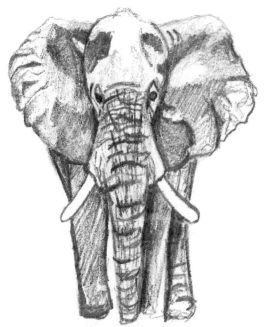

AN ELEPHANT NEVER FORGETS.

Today I got lots of baby cuddles, including with my friend's 3-week-old. I'd got him some elephant-themed gifts as she has always loved elephants. As have I. They are such majestic gentle giants, and I read something about them a while ago, which brought me to tears. When one of their herd dies, they hold a funeral and won't leave the corpse alone for days. They stand and sway and mourn their loved ones. There is something so moving and reassuring about that. There is so much more to the animal kingdom than we understand or give credit for.

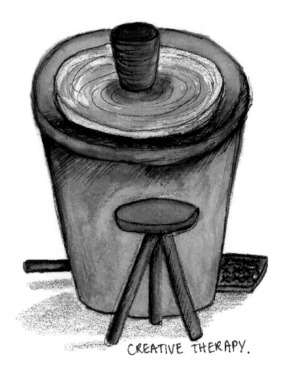

CREATIVE THERAPY.

Today I had an hour to escape to Milland Pottery, run by the very talented Angie, an NCT friend of my Mum. I was feeling pretty stressed on my way there, with treatment day looming tomorrow. I start to get anxiety just thinking about it and even develop nausea as my brain knows what is coming. Anyway, after an hour at Angie's, turning some pots I threw last time then scoring the clay before I paint them next session, I felt like a different person. It is incredible how spending time being creative can affect your mood; I strongly believe this applies to everyone. In fact, I was in such a good mood I belted along with absolute90s the whole way home.

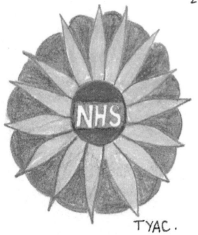

TYAC.

Today was round 4 at the Royal Surrey TYAC, where Sam and Claire took such amazing care of me. We were there for about 4 hours as it was new drugs today; Herceptin was done through an injection in my thigh, then the Dosetaxel, which had to go very slowly through a drip. Finally, I decided to have my PICC line out for a number of reasons, mainly because it's a pain to carry Milo but also because I'm desperate to go swimming. Despite being slightly over the threshold, I feel incredibly lucky to have been invited to the Teen and Young Adult ward. The care is so individualised and personable that I feel like I'm sitting with friends while having my chemo. It makes a world of difference. Thank you TYAC!

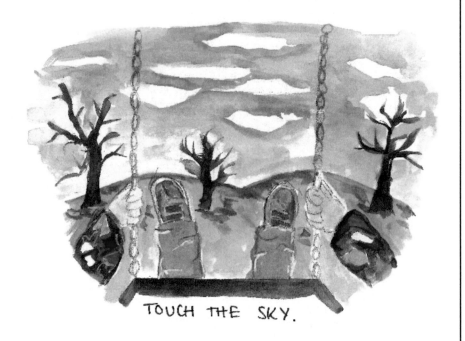

TOUCH THE SKY.

Feeling ok today, not as sicky as the EC, just flu-like symptoms, so hoping that will last. Grandma and Pop pops are here this weekend, so they took Milo out this morning, giving me a chance to rest. Had a little more energy this afternoon, so we all went to the park, and Milo loved the swings. Such a beautiful afternoon of sunshine which makes me so excited for spring.

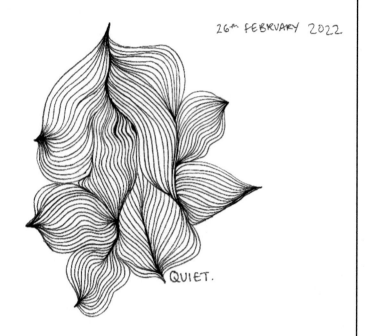

QUIET.

Today was a quiet day. Milo was out with Grandma and Pop pops most of the day so that I could rest. I spent the day lying on the sofa, staring out the window, longing to enjoy the beautiful weather. Days like today are frustrating and lonely. I need the quiet and rest, but I resent the loneliness and feeling like I am wasting a day. Messages of support from friends and family are a comfort, but it's hard not to feel like I'm lying in a deep hole. Thank god this chemo doesn't seem to cause the same level of sickness. Just have to ride out these sleepy days and wait for my energy to return.

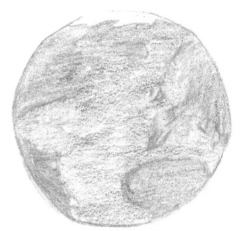

OUR PLANET.

Another quiet day today with low energy levels again. It's hard to motivate yourself to do anything when you feel so weak. Luckily Megs & Nick came over this afternoon with baby Olive so I could have cuddles. I got the photo album out from when Meg & I went travelling back in 2010 and we had a good laugh recounting the ridiculous stories. We were so lucky to go to so many incredible places and meet so many wonderful people on this planet. It makes me think about what is happening in Ukraine. It is heartbreaking and scary, but what gives me faith is the response from people and the support flooding in from all the over the world. Sending all my thoughts and love to the people of Ukraine. Putin and cancer can both fuck off!

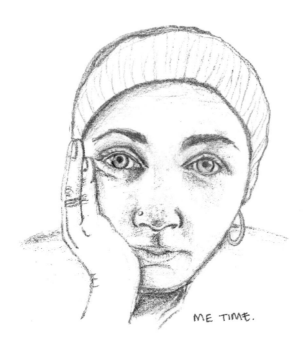

ME TIME.

Being off work means that I have me to keep myself company during the week when most people are at work. Alone time can cause a whole host of anxieties and thought patterns, including feeling like I 'should' be doing more. However, I believe it is important for everyone to give themselves the time and space you need - when you need it. Self-care cannot be put off until tomorrow. Whether it's letting your body repair itself or your mind heal, we all need Me time.

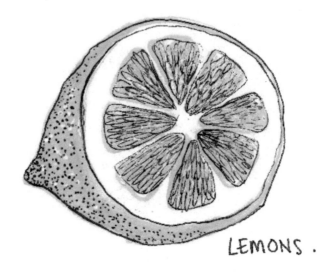

LEMONS .

Happy Pancake day, lovely people. Milo loved mixing the ingredients and then pouring them into the pan but wasn't particularly keen on actually waiting for them to cook, bless him. I had lemon and sugar like I always do. You can't beat the old classic. It was a sugary highlight on a rather sleepy day. And you know what they say about lemons ...

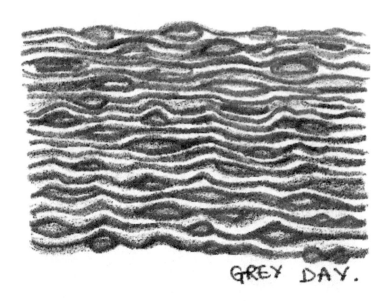

GREY DAY.

My oh my, today was grey. Luckily, I had the morning with baby Charlie and the wonderful Emma. Then this afternoon, it was back to the hospital for an ultrasound to check to see if the chemo was working. The great news is the lump has shrunk, which means the hell my body is going through is actually working! I was absolutely dreading walking into that room as that was the first place I realised something was seriously wrong. But we are making progress and are on our way to kicking cancer's butt. *This is my attempt at drawing an ultrasound, and the first time I went there was a big black hole in the middle where the lump was. It was a relief to see the more normal grey waves today.

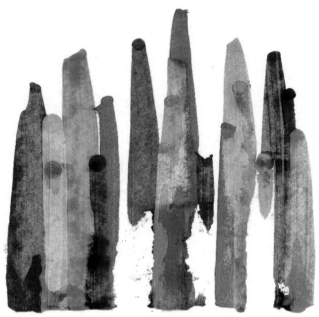

A SPLASH OF COLOUR.

Another grey drizzly day. Made better this afternoon by seeing my cousins who are over from California. God, what I'd do for some of that Californian sunshine. Today's art is so much fun and super easy to create, so if you've got some paint and a shower squeegee at home, have a go! Simply dot the paint around the top, then drag it down et voila.

Dammit Doll

" WHENEVER THINGS DON'T GO SO WELL
AND YOU WANT TO HIT THE WALL AND YELL
HERE'S A LITTLE DAMMIT DOLL
THAT YOU CAN'T DO WITHOUT
JUST GRASP IT FIRMLY BY THE LEGS
AND FIND A PLACE TO SLAM IT!
AND AS YOU WHACK THE STUFFING OUT
YELL DAMMIT, DAMMIT, DAMMIT! "

DAMMITDOLLS.COM

An incredibly apt gift as Milo was testing my patience this morning, and after a few nights of terrible sleep, I was at the end of the rope. My cousins came and took us out for lunch and gave me this 'Dammit Doll,' which is brilliant and would highly recommend for anyone going through treatment... or toddlers... or any stress, in fact, it works a treat. An added bonus is Milo likes whacking it against the furniture so he too can work through his stress!

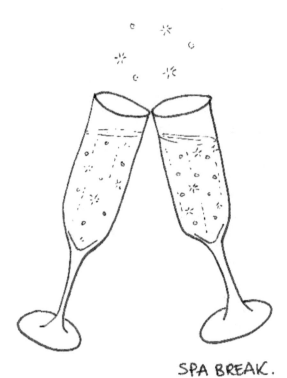

SPA BREAK.

Mum has brought me on a spa break to Champneys, which is simply splendid. After an afternoon of enjoying the steam room, sauna and pool, I had an incredible facial. She was so sweet and used oil combinations that would help with my dry skin and even gave my chemo-chapped hands a special massage. Now we're chilling with a glass of Prosecco in our room before heading to dinner. Feel utterly spoilt by and incredibly grateful for Mama.

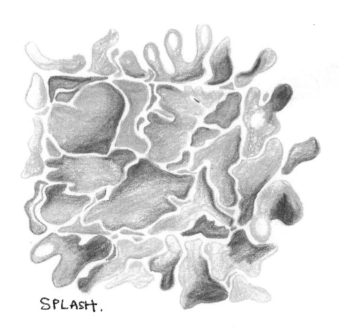

SPLASH.

We stayed at the spa for the morning, and I went for a swim while Mum had a treatment. I have always loved the water and feel a sense of calm whenever swimming. After having my PICC line removed, I couldn't wait to get back in, and today did not disappoint.

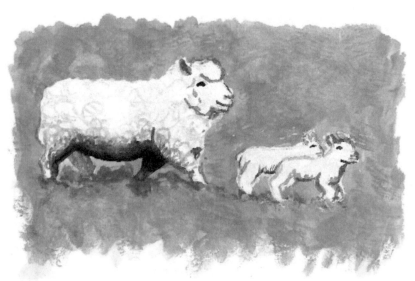

NEW BEGINNINGS.

Wow, what a stunning day. I feel so lucky that I could spend the afternoon out in the sunshine with Milo. He did really well and understood when I said I couldn't carry him, so he'd have to walk the whole thing. We walked past a field of ewes with their little lambs that were so sweet. They are a few weeks old now, so feeling more confident and going off in little groups but would dash back to hide behind their Mums when we walked past.

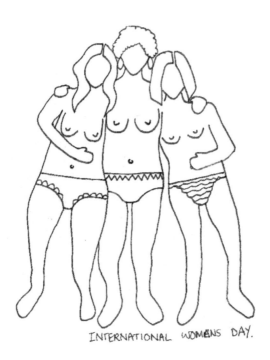

INTERNATIONAL WOMENS DAY.

Happy International Women's Day to all you incredible, beautiful, and brave women out there. Also want to take this opportunity to say, Ladies - know and love your bodies, check yourself regularly, and if something doesn't feel right, whether it be physically or hormonally, then go and see someone and don't take "I'm sure you'll be fine" for an answer. We have to advocate for ourselves in a world where women's health is not a priority.

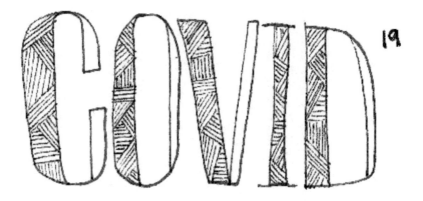

IT FINALLY CAUGHT ME.

After 2 years, COVID has finally caught me. Woke up this morning with a temperature, so rang the hospital, and they told me to come into A&E. When having chemo, your white blood cell count is low, so your body isn't able to fight infection very well so as soon as you get a fever, they want to get you on antibiotics straight away. They took my blood and obviously a COVID test which came back positive. They have put me on fluids and are monitoring me, but they don't seem too worried, which is reassuring. I have a private room in the COVID ward, which is surreal. Hopefully, I will start feeling better and be able to go home tomorrow, missing my team already!

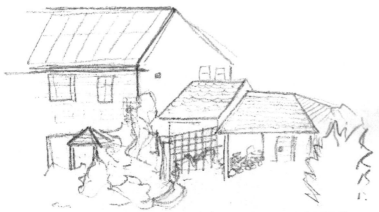

HOME SWEET HOME.

A quick sketch tonight as I'm exhausted but so happy to be home. I was only in the hospital for a day 1/2, but I was really missing home and my fam. The Drs were happy to discharge me as my COVID symptoms aren't too bad, but they have given me antivirals which should help to stop COVID taking its grip. My oncology doctor also put me on antibiotics as a precaution, as it would be pretty serious if I developed an infection. All in all, it's good news, and I was pleased to be told I could come home, even if it was at 9 am and I didn't actually leave until 6 pm. Anyway, so incredibly grateful for the NHS and their care and thanks for all the love and support, as always.

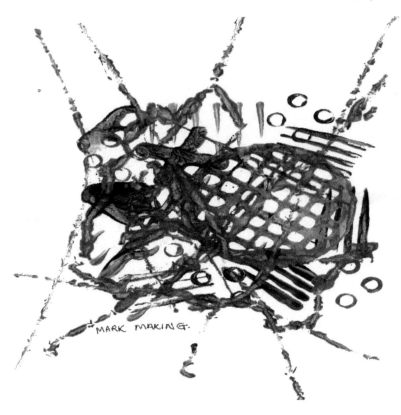

MARK MAKING.

Woke feeling much better after a night in my own bed. The night sweats are still horrible, but I think that's down to menopause again. To be honest, the various side effects and symptoms are all starting to blur together, and I'm not really sure what is causing what... so I've stopped thinking about it. Milo and I went for a very wet walk this afternoon, then decided to have some creative time together when we got back. Mark making is so fun, and Milo loved finding different things to print with.

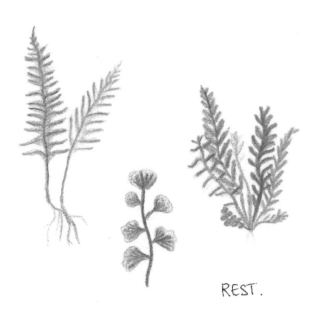

REST.

This is the pattern on the curtains in our living room. It's what I can see from my spot on the sofa, which I've resumed since catching COVID. Today has been bittersweet. I feel better, just exhausted which I am quickly becoming to use to, so we went for a gentle walk in the sunshine. I love having time with my little fam and cherish the memories. However, this weekend we were meant to have friends staying and were planning to go down to the beach for a swim. So it's bittersweet. It's hard not to feel frustrated when my 'good' weekends are taken away from me as the next treatment day looms. So fuck COVID and FUCK cancer.

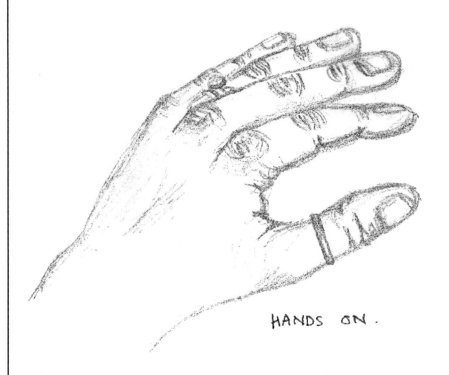

HANDS ON.

One of the strangest side effects of this chemo has been on my hands. It started off with them being super sore and like they were always numb from the cold. Then they started to dry out and become chapped. Sorry to be gross, but the skin has now started peeling off my fingertips, so bizarre. Luckily, I have been gifted with lots of lovely hand cream recently.

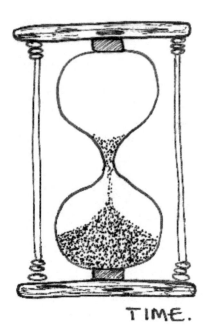

TIME.

At the moment, I constantly swing between wanting time to speed up and then slow down again (something I know we all do a lot of the time.) After having chemo, I wish the time away, waiting till I feel like myself again, then, as I do, I dig my heals in. I desperately try and find the balance between making every minute of "good" time count and not exhausting myself. The tiredness is infuriating, something I've noted a lot of other cancer patients saying. Just have to enjoy the little things, like bath time with Milo this evening.

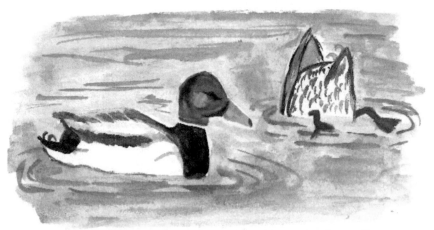

BOTTOMS UP.

Today I got a call from my oncology doctor telling me that due to only just getting over COVID, he doesn't want to go ahead with the planned chemo on Thursday. It was devastating news as, despite the fact I was not looking forward to it at all, it pushed everything back by a week. I have very little control over my life at the moment, and I feel like this has taken away the little I had left, as weekends I had planned between treatments will now be ruined. However, I totally get why and trust that it is the right thing to give my body another week to recover. To not let the day be ruined, I took Milo to the park in the afternoon sunshine; he loved watching the ducks. He particularly enjoyed it when they put their bottoms in the air and wanted to have a go himself.

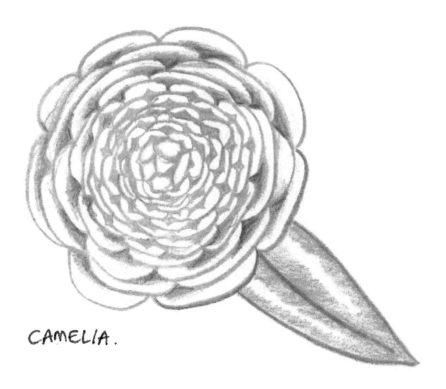

CAMELIA.

Despite the cruddy weather today, I couldn't help but notice the beautiful Camelia that is blooming in our garden. The other blossoms are starting to appear which is delightful and with the sunshine on its way, things are looking up!

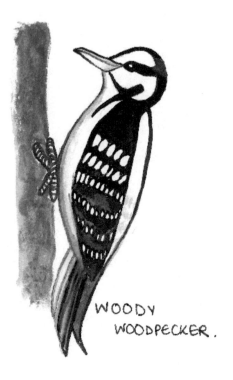

WOODY
WOODPECKER.

There are some woodpeckers that live in the woods behind our house. On our walk this morning, Milo and I could hear them knocking away but couldn't spot them amongst the trees, though we have seen one once or twice. All the birds were in a beautiful chorus this morning, I imagine they're as pleased about the sunshine as I am. Today was meant to be treatment day so I have mixed feelings. Can't quite believe I feel disappointed about not feeling crap right now. However, it does mean we can enjoy the sunshine at the beach tomorrow, so swings and roundabouts, I am coming for you!

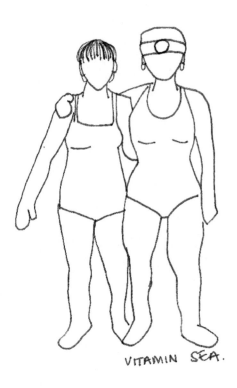

VITAMIN SEA.

Today was a beach day. The weather was incredible and my Dad even drove the campervan down so we could sit and have lunch looking out at the sea. The best part was finally being able to take a very quick dip in the sea with Mum. Part of the reason I enjoy the swim so much is because in that moment, I am in total control of what I am putting my body through.

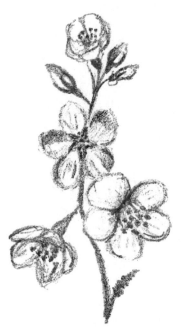

CHERRY BLOSSOM.

Today, Mum and I went to Wisley Garden Centre. The cherry trees were in full blossom and looked astonishing against the bright blue sky. We took milo to the packed out play park before heading off to meet my family for lunch and a walk. One of the things cancer has made me grateful for, other than not having to worry about shaving my armpits which is simply great, is that my appreciation for days like today, which is unmeasurable. I genuinely treasure the memories. Hope everyone had a fabulous Saturday.

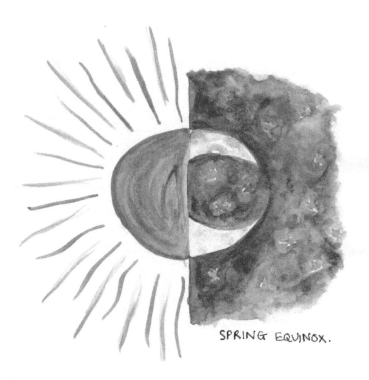

SPRING EQUINOX.

Another beautiful day spent pottering around the house and garden. The weeding has already begun and there are always jobs in the house to do so we were both busy while Milo pottered between us, occasionally very unhelpfully launching something into the pond. Toddlers. The day finished with an MRI (on a Sunday?!) to check my heart function, which I'll find out the results for tomorrow.

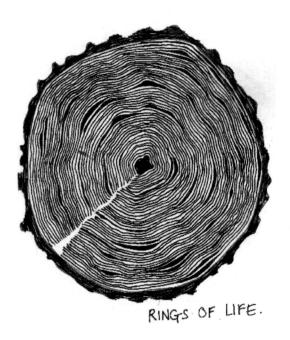

RINGS OF LIFE.

Today, Milo fell asleep on the way back from nursery, so I had to sit in the car with him for a while making sure he was in deep sleep before going inside. As I sat there, I studied the log pile that Harry carefully built and the endless rings in the cut wood. Thought about how in the next winter, this will be our main source of heat with the energy prices going up so dramatically. It just blows my mind how they think people are going to be able to afford to live.

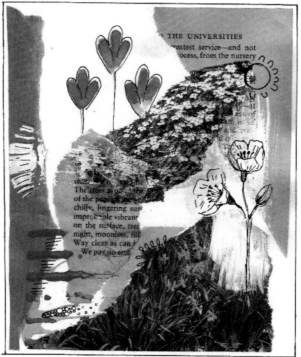

THE GARDEN.

Feeling like myself today and after a lovely walk this morning,
I had some time in my studio to create. The sun was
streaming in and I could hear the bird song while I sat and
felt a sense of calm.

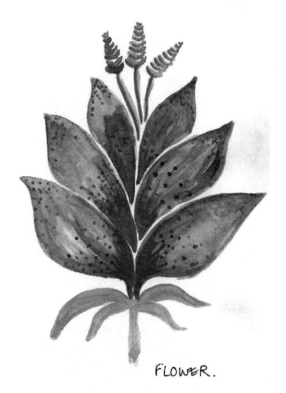

FLOWER.

Today, I feel frustrated. I had my appointment with the oncologist who said that I can go ahead with the next round of chemo. However, he went on to explain that my surgery would most likely be 6-8 weeks after my last round, which is longer than I originally thought. It feels all up in the air and so out of my control which is infuriating. Then to top it off, I found out this afternoon the pharmacy is running behind and my chemo won't be ready for tomorrow so I'll have to have it on Friday instead. I genuinely just have to take a deep breath and try to let it wash over me. I have to trust the process and control the things I still can.

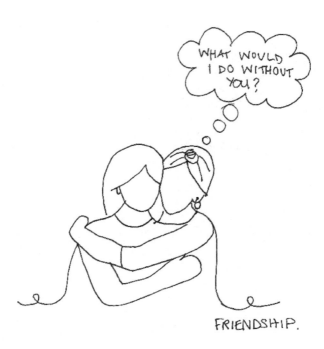

FRIENDSHIP.

This morning, I was feeling low. I don't really know why, possibly drank more more wine than I can muster last night to calm my frustrations or just feeling out of control so my anxiety is creeping in. Either way, I was a tad emotional but took Milo to playgroup then came home. Then had various friends drop in to see me all afternoon with cakes and baby cuddles. It's incredible how your support system can pull you up without having to say anything. Just their company made me feel myself again. So unbelievably grateful for my amazing friends.

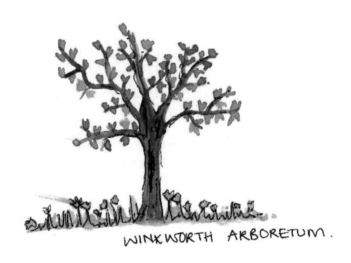

WINKWORTH ARBORETUM.

This morning, Mum and I took Milo to the arboretum to look at all the blossom trees. It was a beautiful morning in a stunning place but I struggled to control my anxiety the closer we got to leaving to go to the hospital. It's been a month since my last treatment so I was dreading it more than the first one. Luckily, Harry was able to come in with me even though I was back in the main ward which was packed. By the time I got in there and got going, I felt better and the 3 1/2 hours passed quickly (helped by beating Harry 35 - 15 in casino). However, I'm now home and the tiredness and aches have started to creep in and it's like a dark cloud descending. Just got to button down the hatches and get through the next week or so. Hope everyone has a lovely weekend, sending love.

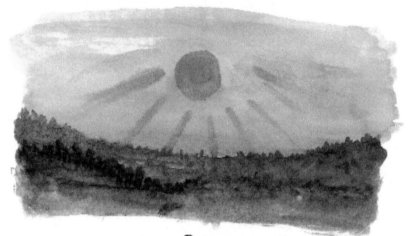

SUNSET WALKS.

What a beautiful day. I was so glad to be able to enjoy some of it and spent the morning in the garden before heading in for a much needed nap. Then this afternoon couldn't resist taking a very slow plod to the pub with my team. We stopped at our sunset spot on the way back and took in the incredible views. So so thankful to have settled here and got this house before this all happened. Feeling very sleepy but grateful.

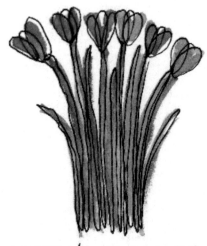

MOTHER'S DAY. ♡

Happy Mother's Day to all the beautiful Mamas out there. To those that look amazing and seem unfaltering. To those that have lost and have suffered beyond belief. To those that are doing everything for their kids and it seems like it's not enough. To those who are still waiting. To those who never were but have mothered their loved ones so ferociously. To those missing their Mum today. Finally, to my own Mama. It's hard to put into words how incredible you have been over the last few months. You have gone above and beyond to help and support us despite the pain this is causing you. You are the most selfless, caring, and strong person I know and I am so proud and grateful to call you my mother. Love you, immeasurably.

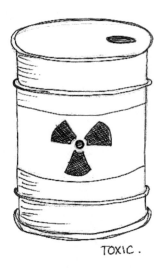

TOXIC .

Before I write today's post, I need to say that I am not doing so in order to gain sympathy but to try and cast a light on how I am feeling. If this in some way helps someone else going through this or in supporting a loved one then it will be worth my crude honesty. Today was hard. I slept terribly and woke feeling sick then spent the day crumpled on the sofa. I feel like shit. I feel like the toxins that were pumped into me. I am drained. I am a drain. I feel like I do nothing but suck the life from those around me just like the cancer is trying to suck the life from me. It's a horrible feeling and like a black cloud hovering, which drenches those around me. I know that they wouldn't have it any other way but the guilt of what this is doing to my loved ones is unbearable. I know that these bad days will pass and as I start to feel better, so will my outlook. But on days like today I'm back to telling cancer to fuck off and stop causing so much pain.

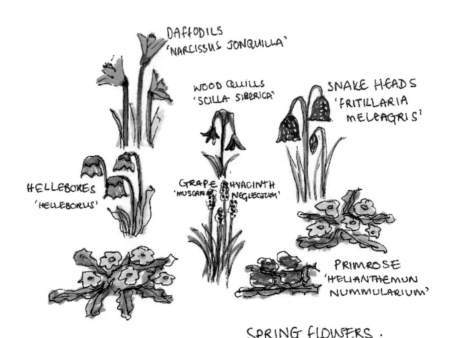

DAFFODILS
'NARCISSUS JONQUILLA'

WOOD QUILLS
'SCILLA SIBERICA'

SNAKE HEADS
'FRITILLARIA MELEAGRIS'

HELLEBORES
'HELLEBORUS'

GRAPE HYACINTH
'MUSCARI NEGLECTUM'

PRIMROSE
'HELIANTHEMUN NUMMULARIUM'

SPRING FLOWERS.

Today was a much better day. Still exhausted with metallic taste in my mouth but managing to eat and actually walk around. Had a quiet morning while Milo was at nursery and had my first counselling session curtesy of the Fountain Centre, which was great to talk out my inner monologue without causing a loved one any more pain. This afternoon, I even managed to get out in the garden for a bit of much needed weeding. The spring flowers were so beautiful and again, I find myself so grateful to have inherited such a stunning garden. Trying to do it justice by learning all the correct names rather than just "yellow flower" or "leafy one."

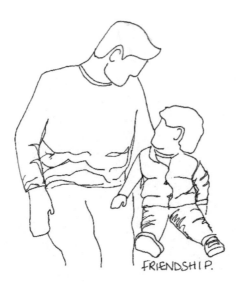

FRIENDSHIP.

Today I felt a little more myself which was a relief. I spent the morning in the studio then we had a visit from Milo's guardian, Rory. I absolutely love the relationship that is blossoming between one of my closest friends and my son. We went for a walk then a play in the park and I'm not sure who enjoyed the playground more. Thank you for visiting Uncle Rory , it was wonderful as always.

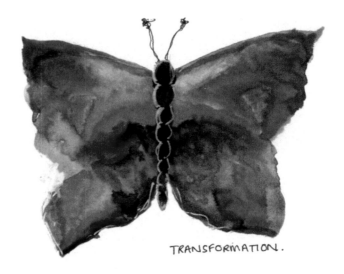

TRANSFORMATION.

One of Milos favourite books at the moment is 'The hungry Caterpillar' of which my favourite part is the butterfly at the end. I've been thinking a lot recently about what is at the end of this journey and getting back to "normal." What I have come to realise is that when going through something, may it be a crappy break up, a pandemic, a terrible loss or a difficult disease, it is not about returning to the old but rather adapting to this new YOU. I have to learn to love my body for what it has become and its betrayals. I'm not implying that there is always a silver lining because let's be honest, sometimes things are just plain crap, but you can still control how you handle things and what you make of your life.

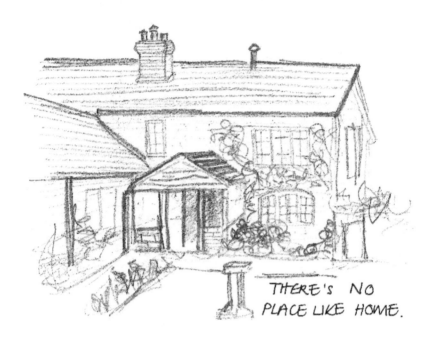

THERE'S NO
PLACE LIKE HOME.

Today is Mum's birthday so we are all at home for the
weekend. I love it when we are all back here together, eating
and drinking too much, going for long walks and arguing over
board games. It's mayhem but simply perfect.

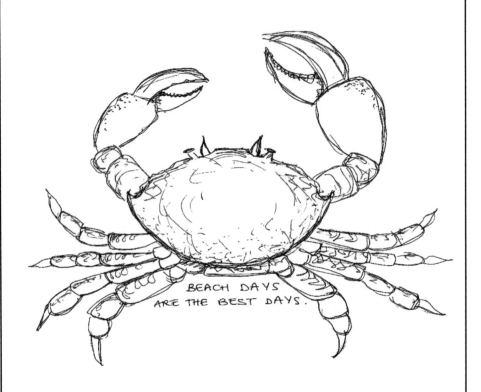

BEACH DAYS
ARE THE BEST DAYS.

A family day at the beach today. The weather was beautiful but the occasional artic gust kept us out of the sea this time. However, we did manage a little picnic in a sheltered spot which was so lovely and felt like a special treat. There were lots of crab shells washed up so my brother gave them to Milo who was on his shoulders, who then proceeded to crush them into his hair. Little monkey. The most wonderful memories to treasure.

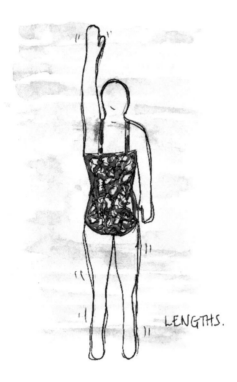

LENGTHS.

After an amazing weekend with the family, we spent the evening at the spa. It was so lovely to get back in the pool and I challenged myself to swim 10 lengths. After only 4, my legs were cramping and I was tempted to give up and head back to the steam room but I persevered and felt pleased to complete my little challenge. I have been motivated by Adele Roberts who has been running through her chemo. It's frustrating to feel so unfit but I know it's temporary and part of the journey.

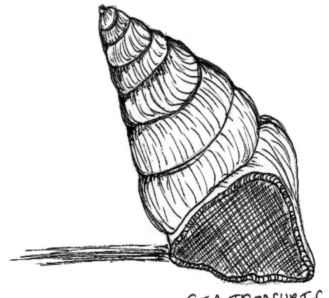

SEA TREASURES.

Back to the seaside today with the gorgeous Emma Pickett.
We had breakfast in the cafe and watched the stormy waves
with trepidation. With full bellies, we stepped out the door
onto the pebble beach to make a decision.... We were going in!! A
quick change and we made our way down to the water's edge.
By far, my coldest swim so far, I didn't even manage any
strokes just waded out to waist height and dunked. Bladdy
freezing. But bladdy exhilarating at the same time. On our
way back up, Emma picked up some little shells as a souvenir of
our cold swim.

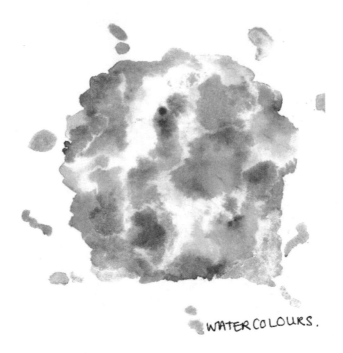

WATER COLOURS.

Today was another good day, starting with my second counselling session. I was less teary today, probably due to not recently having chemo and feeling like crap. So it was good to be able to work through some things and get out some thoughts that have been stuck and going round my head. Then I had a lovely visit from friends for coffee before Milo's grandma arrived. We had a nice afternoon exploring Waggoners Wells followed by a special treat in the pub. So glad it's getting my warm (again). Bring on the sunshine!

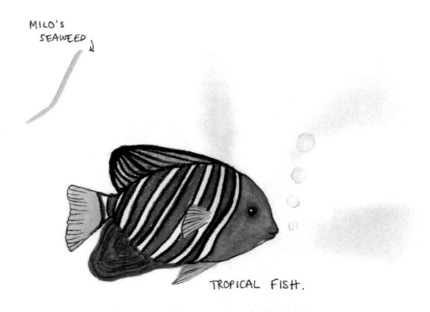

MILO'S
SEAWEED

TROPICAL FISH.

Another lovely day with Milo and Grandma. I spent time in the
studio this morning after receiving a reply to my application to
an Art Therapy Masters to say that I got an interview.
I've got a couple of weeks to prepare, so need to get my
academic brain back on and remember how to write a sentence
that doesn't include "I"?! Then this afternoon, we took Milo
to Little Street before going into the outdoor shop where Milo
enjoyed running in and out of the tents and looking at all the
tropical fish.

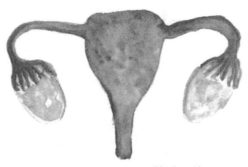

FERTILTY.

Today, I was in the hospital to get my Zoladex injection. The first time was horrible as the needle is stupidly big but since then, I apply a little numbing cream which helps ease the pain. I have to have the injection once a month to suppress my ovaries in order to protect them from the chemo. One of the biggest upsets when I got my diagnosis was the realisation that we won't be having a baby any time soon. We had planned to start trying for our second this year so it was a bit of a shock. I understand how lucky I am to have Milo but it was still devastating to know that there will be such a big age gap. I had an appointment with the gynaecologist and we discussed freezing eggs but the whole process seemed too risky. In order to collect the eggs, they would have to wait for a cycle which would have delayed my chemo starting and they would have had to inject me with oestrogen, which would have helped the cancer to grow. I have to go onto tamoxafen for two years once I have finished treatment then we can try again. The doctor was very optimistic about our chances of getting pregnant again in a few years so we made the decision to get me well without delay. I know of so many women who have cancer and now infertile so I know how lucky I am to have the possibility of being pregnant again one day. And if not, there are others options we will have to explore in order to grow our family. For now, it's perfect the way it is.

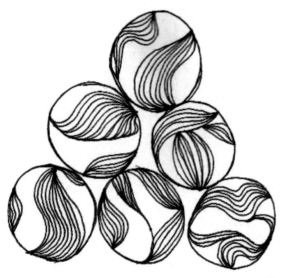

LOST ME MARBLES.

Milo's favourite toy for the last few weeks has been the marble run. We have got the building down to a fine art and constructed a tower where the marbles spiral round then fall straight back into the tin ready to be plucked out and dropped down again. It is simply addictive and I find myself getting completely immersed in the play. I don't know if it's the hours spent at home and not working or that marbles are just awesome but I do feel like I've got slightly mad. Ahh well, might as well embrace it now.

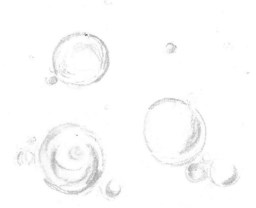

BUBBLES.

I sat for ages this evening, pencil poised above the page with absolutely no idea what to draw. We've had a wonderful day and been very busy with a lovely walk to the pub this afternoon. I even put a cheeky bet on the grand national and won a little! This evening, I am totally wiped and had no energy to draw, then I heard Milo screaming in the bathroom down so went to help with bath time and distracted him by blowing bubbles in my hands just like my Dad used to do.

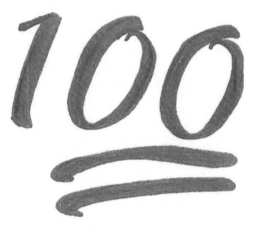

THE BEST KIND OF SUNDAY.

Today was my favourite kind of Sunday. Beautiful weather and a walk to the pub with friends to sit in the garden with chips and a beer. Then the afternoon was spent in the garden, weeding and mowing before having our first BBQ of the season. Also today is my 100th post. When I started this project, I wasn't sure how long I would keep it up and whether I would find it helpful. What has actually happened has been incredible. I have felt love and support not only from friends and family but people from all over the world. There are days when I really don't have the energy or feel narcissistic, but the lovely messages I've received over the last few months have made it all worth it. You guys are the best and I'm so glad to have you all in this journey with me.

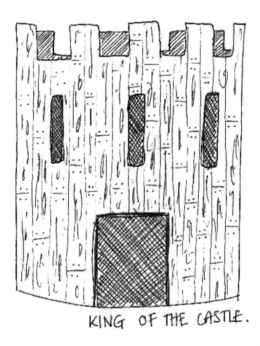

KING OF THE CASTLE.

After a relaxing morning with Mum at her health club, this afternoon I took Milo to meet Nikki and Jesse at the park. There was a little turret there which Milo loved climbing to the top of as his favourite song at the moment is, "I'm the king of the castle..." which he gets very cross at me if I sing and says, "No, I am the King." No surprise there. On days like this, I feel like the king of the castle but as treatment day looms I know I'll feel like the Dirty rascal by the end of the week. However, knowing this is the penultimate round is definitely getting me a little excited ... bring it on!

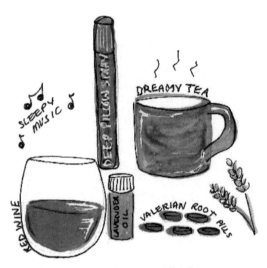

INSOMNIA.

Sleep is a bizarre thing. I've never been very good at it and have struggled with insomnia and sleep anxiety for most of my life. It comes and goes, but on the whole, I've been lucky and since getting my anxiety under control, I've been able to sleep well without many aids. Since my diagnosis, it's been touch and go. You'd think feeling exhausted all day means you sleep like a log but nooo. Some nights are fine but some are torture. Your brain won't switch off, your heart races and you just can't get to the right temperature. Whether its the side effects of the chemo, the menopause or just knowing there is a war going on inside my body, insomnia sucks. I use various things to help, some doctor recommended, some definitely not. But hey ho, whatever works right?

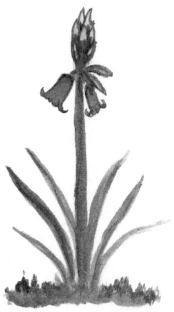

BLUEBELLS.

Most days we walk in the woods behind our house and I love watching them change with the seasons. The bluebells are starting to bloom which will leave a carpet of purple on the forest floor like something out of a fairy tale. It's magical. It makes me excited for what is to come. Tomorrow is my penultimate chemo and bizarrely I feel excited as it means I only have one left after that. One more round of drugs before I am onto the next stage of surgery. One more step towards ridding myself of this monster!

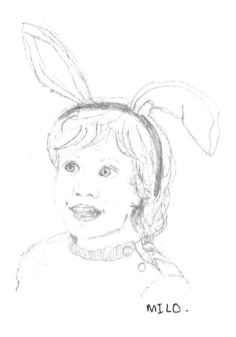

MILO.

I sat down with Milo while he was having tea and asked him what I should draw today, to which he replied, "Milo." So as per most of his requests, no matter how ridiculous, I obliged. He is my absolute favourite and gives me the purpose I need at the moment being off work. He certainly challenges me on a daily basis but never fails to make me laugh and melts my heart when he rubs my back and says, "How are you feeling Mummy?" Today was my 6th dose and it went surprisingly quickly. The nurses were amazing and made me feel so welcome and comfortable, like being part of a family. Only one more infusion to go, yippee! And it's bank holiday weekend so we're off for a few days down to Dorset in the campervan, which we are all far too excited about.

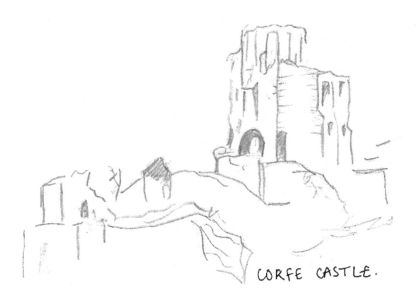

CORFE CASTLE.

Quick sketch by torch light this evening as we got back late from our visit to our favourite pub down here, the Scott's Arms. We spent the morning travelling down to Dorset and parked up the camper in the sunshine. The walk up to the pub was pretty muddy but the views were incredible and there were lots of tiny baby lambs hopping about. Jerk chicken and a Red stripe (for H, just water for me at the moment) for dinner then a quick march back down the hill at the sunset. We bundled Milo on bed and are now huddled in our awning. I feel surprisingly okay after yesterday's treatment, just making sure to drink lots and take it easy.

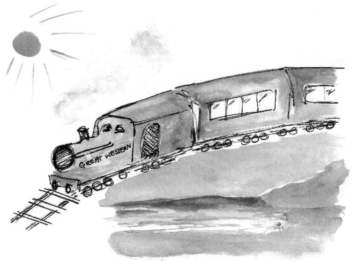

A TRAIN RIDE TO THE BEACH.

Today we took Milo on his very first train ride, which was pretty damn special. He loved every minute and watching the amazement on his face was magical. We sat on the beach and had our sandwiches and chips followed by a delicious ice cream. I had little dozes throughout the day which kept me going. It's amazing to be able to enjoy the bank holiday weekend with my little family and I'm so thankful.

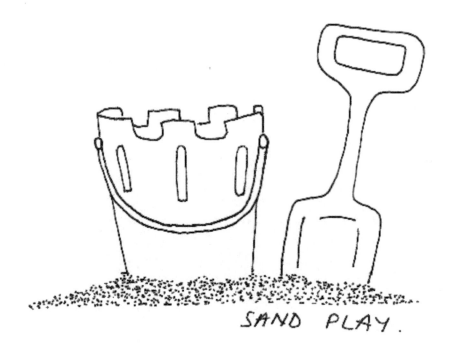

SAND PLAY.

Spent the day at Studland Bay today, which is one of our favs. My brother and family arrived last night so Milo and his cousin loved playing in the sand with their diggers. Though the sun was shining, the wind was pretty chilly so I sat huddled under a blanket most of the time. Seem to be unable to get myself warm at the moment, not sure if it's the lack of hair or a side effect of chemo, just feel constantly shivery. Though, well worth it to watch the others rolling around in the sand and listen to the crashing waves.

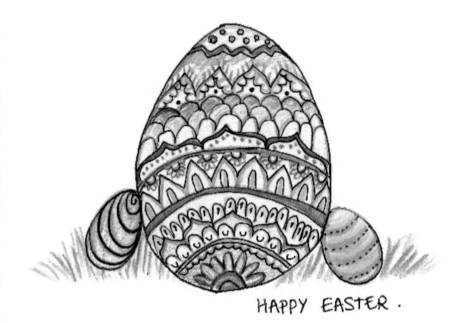

HAPPY EASTER.

After a slow morning of packing up, we set off homeward bound and arrived back to unload the van again this end. Once done, I sat down on the sofa and almost burst into tears from sheer exhaustion. My body feels bruised like it has been on a third day obstacle course and my joints ache like I'm a ninety year old. It was frustrating not having the energy to play but I have to be grateful that I was able to go away this weekend and enjoy being with my family. This week will have to be set aside for recovery but it was so worth it.

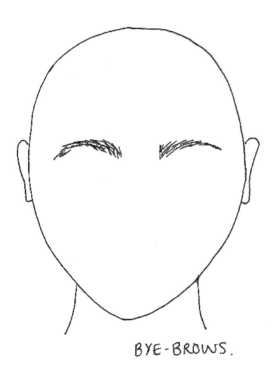

BYE-BROWS.

My eyebrows have finally started to fall out. They haven't completely gone yet but I don't think it'll be long. I've always been lucky to have thick, dark eyebrows so haven't had to think about styling them just tweezing occasionally. I've never been great at makeup (blue eyeshadow was a favourite back in the day) but will have to learn how to fill in the holes above my eyes so I look less like an alien.

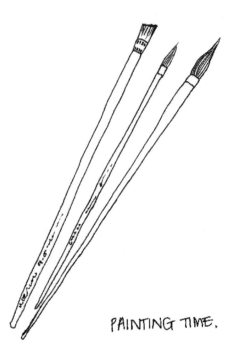

PAINTING TIME.

Still feel pretty exhausted and achy today so I took it easy.
Did manage to get in the studio this afternoon to work on my
self-portrait. I have never painted one before but thought
now was a better time than ever.

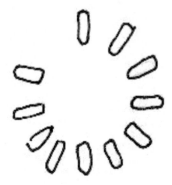

LOADING...

Started the day feeling really fed up. I get angry every time I catch my reflection because I don't see me staring back. I feel stuck in a strange limbo. A space in between. Completely lost. Luckily, my wonderful Mum was on hand to help with Milo so I could rest and the day ended in the loveliest way with old friends and kids in the sunshine eating home-made pizza. I also had an amazing chat with my counsellor tonight and got a lot off my chest. On to the next, keep on plodding.

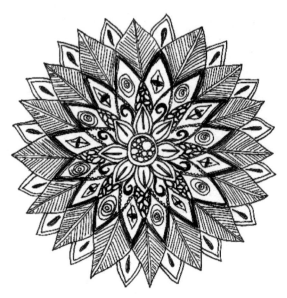

MINDFULLNESS.

We have been talking a lot about Mindfullness recently and how important it is to take stock. I'm trying to practise what I preach and when my mind starts to do cartwheels, I focus on my surroundings and things as simple as the sound of an aeroplane overhead or the feel of the sun on my face. A little of this awareness filtering in and becoming part of your everyday thoughts makes the world of difference to mental health.

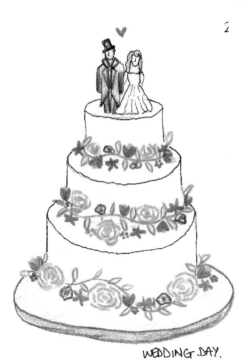

WEDDING DAY.

At a BEAUTIFUL wedding today of our lovely friends who have waited two long years for this day after covid interfered. It feels strange to be dressed up but enjoying drinking, eating, and chatting without thinking about things. Milo is spending the day with his awesome Aunty Tara and cousins, so I can relax and enjoy the party.

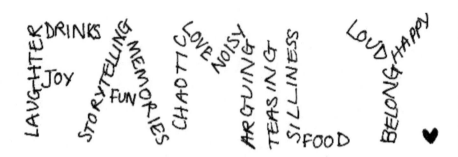

FAMILY.

LAUGHTER DRINKS STORYTELLING MEMORIES CHAOTIC LOVE NOISY ARGUING TEASING SILLINESS FOOD LOUD BELONG HAPPY JOY FUN

THE IN-LAWS.

Woke up feeling pretty sketchy from the wedding but was
whisked off to the spa by my gorgeous sister in law who
spoiled me with a treatment and a relax in the outdoor hot
tub. Felt much better and ready for Poppops birthday lunch
for his 60th. Most of the James crew were there and it was
the usual cacophony of madness which I love. Milo loved playing
with his cousins and running round in the sunshine. Feel so lucky
to have such a wonderful, caring second family.

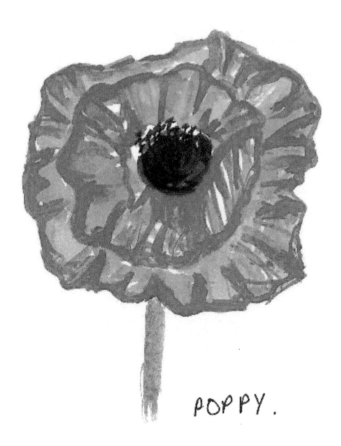

POPPY.

The garden is getting better and better and these gorgeous poppies by the front door catch my eye and always make me smile.

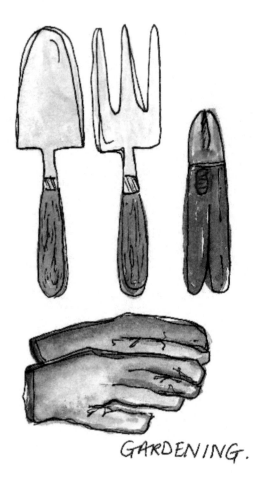

GARDENING.

Now that the weather is warming up, the garden is exploding and I find myself going round and round the same areas trying to keep on top of it. It's like the forth bridge. Milo likes to "help" which is more of a hindrance most of the time but sometimes there are moments where we are digging up weeds together, laughing at the worms and all I want to is freeze time and extend these little moments forever.

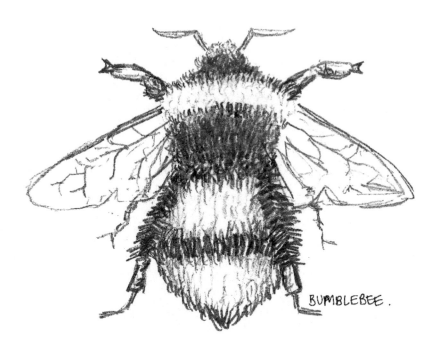

BUMBLEBEE.

On our way up for bath time, we found a bee on the stairs. I scooped it up gently and popped it outside then made a little bowl of sugar water. It looked completely exhausted... know how it feels.

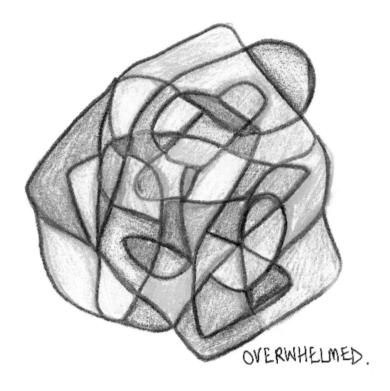

OVERWHELMED.

Today, I had an appointment with my consultant about my surgery. It was only half an hour but felt like four days worth of information and came away feeling totally overwhelmed. My brain was scrambled and felt like I had a panic attack trying to process it all. I took some time out and calmed myself before coming home and having a lovely afternoon with my fam. Was also thinking... you can be overwhelmed and underwhelmed but not just whelmed?

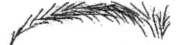 

HI - BROWS.

After seeing something on insta, I ordered some temporary tattoo stick on eye brows and tried them out. I can't quite believe how real they look and I can't quite put into words how much better they make me feel. Losing my eyebrows was way worse than my hair. Felt like I lost a huge part of my identity which was hard and bizarre. Speaking to my counsellor apparently everyone says the same. Who knew ey? Anyway, for anyone who sees this in the same position or knows someone, I highly recommend these as a replacement. I got mine on Etsy but there are loads on Amazon, etc.

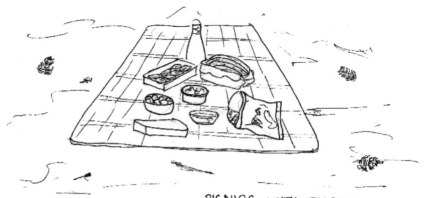

PICNICS WITH FRIENDS.

Had the most wonderful day with our gorgeous friends at
Frensham Little pond. After a delicious picnic, we had a swim
then sat in the sunshine while Milo played in the sand.
Heavenly.

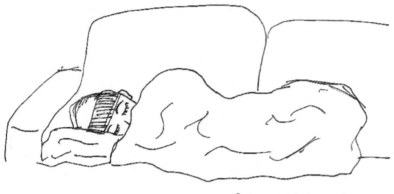

SUNDAY IS FOR REST.

After a busy weekend, I had to surrender myself to the sofa.
Rest is part of this journey as much as positivity is.

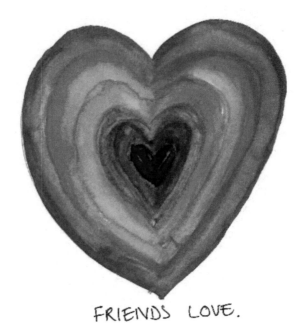

FRIENDS LOVE.

Today, we had our amazing friends over for a BBQ which was so fun. I tried to paint a picture to represent my love for these people and this is what came out. Warm, colourful, fuzzy love for some of my favourite people on this planet. Now, it's time to put our feet up and chiiiiiill.

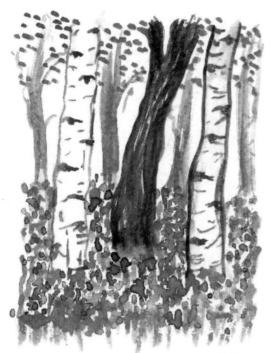

UP IN THE WOODS.

"I'm up in the woods, I'm down on my mind. I'm building a still,
to slow down the time."

Milo and I went for a walk in the bluebell woods today and I
couldn't get this song out of my head. With my last treatment
fast approaching, I have mixed feelings and find myself
digging my heals in. Obviously the fact that it is the last one
is amazing but the thought of feeling all those side effects
again isn't appealing. However, it is the last time then on to
the next part of this journey.

131

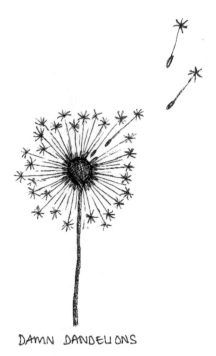

DAMN DANDELIONS

Back in the garden this afternoon trying to get on top of the weeds, especially the dandelions which seem to be popping up everywhere. I try to catch them before they turn to this stage and spread themselves even further. It's on theme of my day really as it involved dashing up to the hospital after speaking to my oncologist who had called to explain my white blood cell count, which was borderline. She said that it was okay to go ahead with chemo as long as I was feeling okay but I needed to have a couple of injections and would have to wait until Friday. Though it's a pain and not what I was expecting, it's definitely preferable to delaying it a week. If I wasn't flexible before, I certainly am learning to be now!

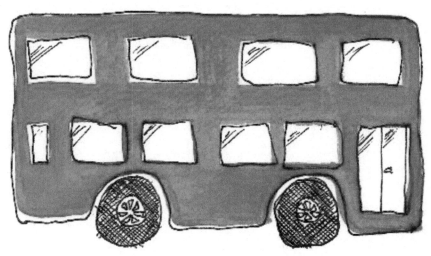

THE BIG RED BUS.

My gorgeous sister in law, Kathryn, arrived today to help look after Milo. He spent the day running around with his cousin, Wilbo, in the garden. On the whole they got on swimmingly though there were arguments over who was playing with the bus. I mean, they didn't care about it last time, but this time it was the holy grail. Anyway, it was an amazing distraction as I barely thought about tomorrow and the last treatment. It seems that excitement is the strongest emotion this evening as I am finally accepting (after being told by many) that it is a milestone and I should be glad to have made it through the last few months. Quite simply could not have done it without my support system for who I am eternally grateful. Let's do this.

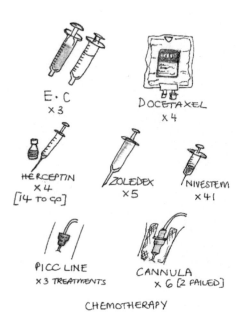

E·C
×3

DOCETAXEL
×4

HERCEPTIN
×4
[14 TO GO]

ZOLEDEX
×5

NIVESTEM
×41

PICC LINE
×3 TREATMENTS

CANNULA
×6 [2 FAILED]

CHEMOTHERAPY

And it's done. Seven rounds of chemotherapy and this is me. I feel relieved that this part of my journey is over for now. I still have fourteen rounds of Herceptin but the side effects of that are manageable. As I left the hospital, I could actually feel the wind in my little baby hairs and I felt like I could let my breath out that I didn't even realise I was holding. This may look like a lot to some and a mere fraction of what others have to go through but this was my experience of chemotherapy and I am glad it's over. Thank you all for the love and support, I genuinely could not have gotten through the last four months without it.

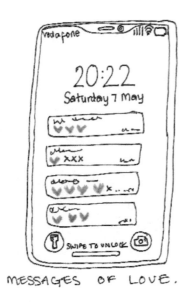

MESSAGES OF LOVE.

I have been completely overwhelmed by the messages of love
and encouragement I have received since my post yesterday.
If I didn't think of it as an achievement before I certainly do
now and though, it still hasn't really sunk in that I have
cancer, I feel proud of where I've got to. If you'd asked me
before I was diagnosed if I could have coped with something
like this, I would probably have said, no way. But it is
incredible what you can manage when you have an amazing
support system and brilliant health care team. As the saying
goes, "You are stronger than you think." The first stage is
over with surgery in a few weeks, but for now I'm going to
give my body and mind time to recover. Big love to you all.

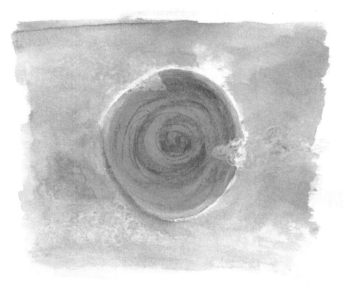

A DAY OF SUNSHINE.

We spent the day in the garden today as different friends dropped by. It was so lovely to be sitting in the sun surrounded by wonderful people, distracting me from how I am feeling. Unfortunately, it has descended this evening and I'm back on the sofa feeling exhausted. However, it has been a fabulous weekend and I'm feeling very loved and looked after.

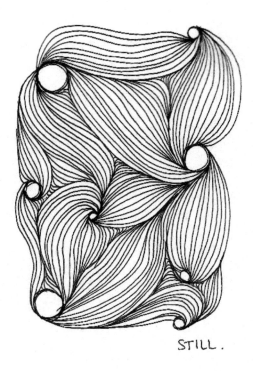

STILL.

After such a busy weekend, today has been a total wipeout.
Mum took Milo so that I could sleep which was very much
needed. As the various side effects sneak back in, I have to
keep reminding myself that it's for the last time.

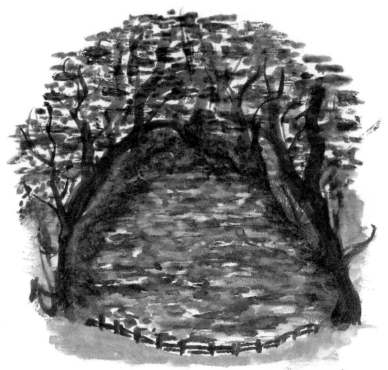

WAGGONERS WELLS.

Today, Milo decided not to nap (toddler Mamas, ya feel the pain?) so we went to Waggoners Wells and spent a dreamy afternoon exploring the ponds in the woods. I have really struggled with headaches today so chucking back the paracetamol but doesn't seem to be keeping them at bay. Maybe a glass of wine will help?!

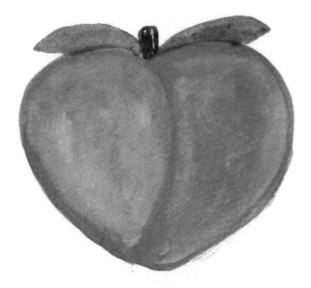

#NOBUTTS

Today's painting is dedicated to the incredible Deborah James who has set up the Bowelbabefund, and in only three days has raised over £3million already. This really is a credit to how many people love and adore her and the impact she has had on everyone's lives, not just those affected by cancer. Her positivity and strength has inspired me in many ways and the work she has done in the cancer world will be her legacy. I hope she can now enjoy her much deserved quiet time surrounded by her loved ones.

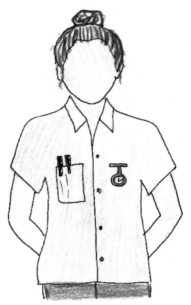

HAPPY INTERNATIONAL NURSES DAY.

Today's post is dedicated to my best friend Meg and all the other incredible nurses out there. I have been so lucky to have such a wonderful care from the nurses on Royal Surrey TYAC and those on Chilworth ward. It takes a certain type of person to dedicate their life to looking after others - caring, selfless, and compassionate to name a few. What on earth would we do without nurses? Thank you all. When Milo saw this and I said it was Meg, he said, "she makes people better."

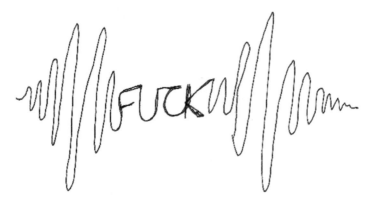

HOSPITAL.

Woke up this morning feeling really rubbish. The last few days I have noticed I have been getting worse rather than better, but today was too much. After calling the chemo hotline, they advised I should come into A&E as I had signs of an infection. My heart rate was through the roof and I had pain in my neck as well as feeling shivery. Sure enough, the bloods came back and my white blood cell count is super low so they have admitted me to the ward. I'm on antibiotics and fluids so fingers crossed I feel better soon. It's so frustrating, especially the fact that it was the last round of chemo and I thought I wouldn't be back here for a while. Have struggled today, feeling crap and not being at home but a little better this evening and very grateful to everyone at Royal Surrey Hospital for how quickly they saw to me and got me looked after.

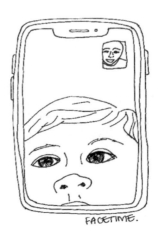

FACETIME.

Today was a pretty slow day. I didn't sleep particularly well being hooked up to the drip all night but woke up feeling a little better. Apart from the nurses popping in to give me my antibiotics and other medication, I'm basically on my own so I am unbelievably thankful for FaceTime. I'm missing Milo ridiculous amounts so being able to play a game of hide and seek with him and my Mum this afternoon really made my day. Milo held onto the phone as he ran round the house hiding in various obvious spots so I got to giggle with him as he waited for his Nanna to find him. Then when it was his turn, I could help him count "1,2,14,19!" then help find her and got to experience the pure and innocent joy of this game. Priceless. Also got a little visit from Harry which was nice. Just got to give myself the time to recover properly and the doctor said that I may be able to go home tomorrow, if not It'll be Monday. Luckily, I've got iplayer on my phone so I will be binging Gavin and Stacey. Thank you for all the love and support.

HYDRATION.

Today, I have been trying really hard to drink a lot of water after the doctor said my electrolytes were down. However, my body still needs a little extra help so I'm back on the drip this evening. The doctor came in earlier and said that my white blood call count is up which is great but she is concerned that I am still dehydrated and have a high heart rate. She did give me the choice and said she could try and get me home tonight but I chose to stay. If you'd told me three days ago that would have been my choice, I would have laughed but I have come to realise that I need to listen to my body and what it's asking for is a break. I know that I have not been giving myself enough time to rest over the last few weeks and if I'm honest, on Friday in A&E was the first time, I felt really sick and it scared me. So as much as I would love to be at home in my own bed, I need to give my body a little more time to heal and mend itself before I go home. I miss Milo ridiculously and it's hard to see him upset on FT but I will make it up in cuddles tomorrow. Hope everyone has had a lovey weekend!

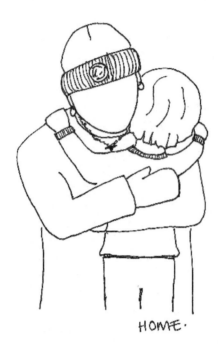

HOME.

After a long day of waiting to be discharged, Mum arrived to keep me company for the last bit. We were told the meds were on their way for about an hour and a half. I was watching the clock and wringing my hands as it crept to Milo's bedtime. All I wanted was a cuddle before he went down. Eventually they agreed to let me go without the discharge letter which they couldn't get hold of and I practically ran out of the hospital and Mum drove us home. As we pulled into the drive, Milo was waving from the bedroom window and I immediately welled up. The hug with him was quite simply the best thing in the world. It's only been four days but the last 24 hours has been torture. It's so good to be home, now time to rest some more.

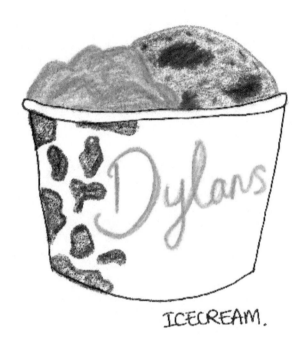

ICECREAM.

After a quiet morning while Milo was at nursery, Grandma and I decided to take Milo for ice cream this afternoon. It was unbelievably yummy and Milo barely said a word while he tucked in. Then we went to the toy shop to get some presents which was a nightmare as he wanted to buy EVERYTHING.

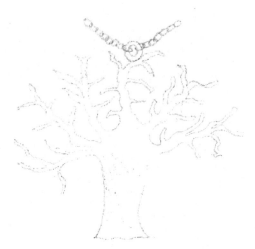

FAMILY.

Today's drawing is of the necklace I gave my mother in law on the day Harry and I got married. It came with a poem about joining the Family Tree and she's worn it ever since as she says she's got us all with her. While I was in hospital, Sarah drove 3hrs 1/2 down to ours to help out. She's spent the week ferrying Milo back and forth to nursery, walking Moose and cleaning the house. It's been lovely to see Milo spend so much 1:1 time with his Grandma and I have no idea how I would have survived this week without her.

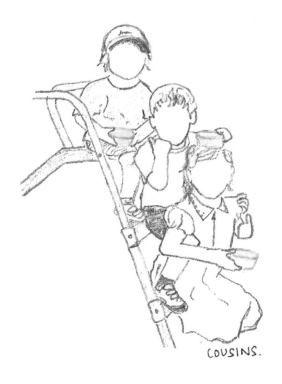

COUSINS.

Today, we drove up to Harry's parents in Warwickshire and picked Milo's cousins up from school. When we got back to the house, we gave them each a bowl of fruit for snack and they all wandered outside. They sat down on the steps of the slide and Sarah managed to capture this gorgeous photo. They are all looking at the camera and grinning ear to ear (whenever I draw faces they end up looking like clowns ,sorry!). They spent the rest of the afternoon running around the garden together before wolfing down a BBQ. It's times like these that are so precious and I value so highly, even more so than before.

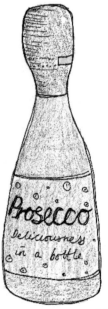

A LITTLE TREAT.

Feeling a little more myself each day and it's an absolute relief to know that this is the last climb and I don't have to sink back down into chemo canyon again. It's been a lovey day with Milo and his cousins. As we put them down this evening, Tara offered me a mini bottle of Prosecco. I haven't drunk for a while so I decided to treat myself and man oh man, is it delicious. Feels so good to be able to enjoy the simple things again.

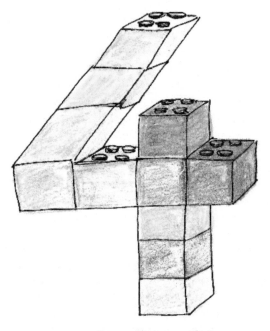

BIRTHDAY BOY.

Today was our nephew Bobby's 4th birthday and it was so lovely. Turns out, being 4 is a big flex (for a 4 year old). Milo loved the bouncy castle and all the cake. The sun was shining and at some point, water balloons came out which had everyone in hysterics. We finished the day by stopping at Pizza Express on the drive home which was a real treat. Exhausted but so content.

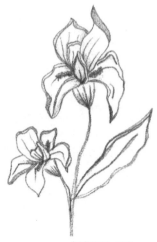

BEARDED IRIS.

Today, some of Harry's family came to visit so we went out for lunch at our favourite pub nearby. It was absolutely delicious and Milo was on great form. After, everyone came back to the house and we spent a while walking round the garden admiring everything that's in bloom. The favourite seemed to be the 'Bearded Iris' which is exquisite. Tonight, I feel hopeful. For the first time in a while I don't feel poorly and I'm starting to really feel there is light at the end of the tunnel.

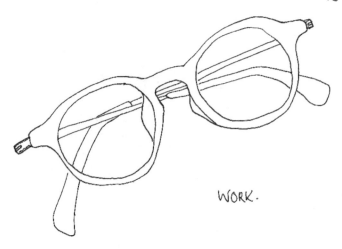

WORK.

Today, while tidying the studio I found my work bag which I haven't touched since I left work the day I found out I had cancer. The notebook is set up for the academic year but stops abruptly in November. I experienced a stab of pain as I rifled through it, envisioning how the year should have been and found my glasses under a folder, which I haven't needed recently. Not working has been hard, a lack of purpose (other than my own health needs) plagues me and I feel at a loss a lot of the time. Though, I am looking to change my career and exciting things lay ahead. Ironically, Harry arrived home from work moaning about his work day, which prompted a 2 hour conversation (accompanied by a bottle of wine) about careers and working. We've concluded that life is far too short to not at least enjoy what you do (obviously we are very aware finances play a huge role) and hopefully we can both find something which allows us to live in this amazing house but also have time to enjoy it.

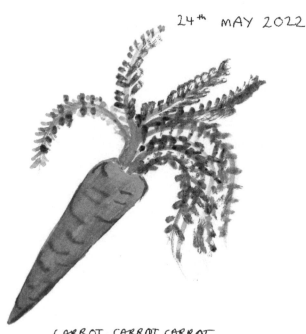

CARROT, CARROT, CARROT.

When I picked up Milo from nursery today, the teacher came out to tell me that he may have a funny tummy as he ate two raw biscuits that were waiting to go in the oven. She had turned away for one second and when she turned back, Milo was stuffing the cookie dough into his mouth. When I looked at him, he was grinning ear to ear as he clutched a funny shaped baked biscuit in his hand. When I asked what it was, he replied "a carrot Mummy".. of course. My brain then started chanting carrot which is a stored memory from my school days and my oldest pal, Ella. She has come to see us this evening and I asked her what the story was behind chanting carrot, which used to send us into hysterics and neither of us can remember. Which if I'm honest, makes it even funnier.

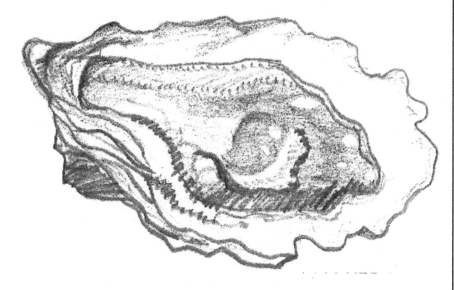

OYSTERS.

Tonight, Harry and I are going for dinner at Moma, the same restaurant we went to just before I started chemo. It feels right to go there to celebrate finishing. Last time we had oysters and I have been thinking about them since, excited for the day when I'd be able to enjoy them again (with an ulcer free mouth).

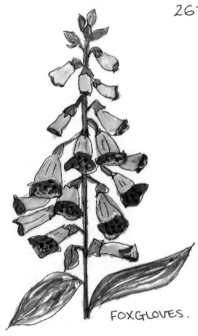

FOXGLOVES.

Today, Mum and I got to visit the Chelsea Flower Show curtesy of my uncle in law, the very talented Joe Swift. It was a real treat to see all the beautiful gardens and displays, and we even got to sit on a couple which was lovely though a little like being on exhibit in the zoo... Joe's garden was stunning and filled with pollinator friendly flowers which were appropriately covered in buzzing bees. Their favourite (and mine) seemed to be the towering, regal foxgloves.

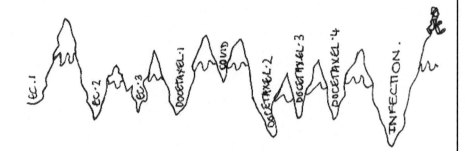

CLIMBING MOUNTAINS.

The last few months have been a series of peaks and troughs.
Some ascents have been harder than others but the hardest
by far is the anticipation of heading down again. The next
stage of this journey is surgery and the first is fast
approaching. I've been riding high on finishing chemo but now
that appointments about the next step have started, I can
feel myself slipping downwards. The only comfort is every step
is one step closer.

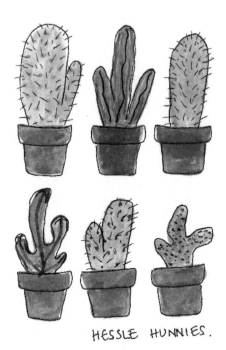

HESSLE HUNNIES.

Today, me and my uni girls had a reunion after two long years,
I lived with these gorgeous girls in Leeds in '6 Hessle View'
and have loved them dearly for over ten years. They never fail
to have me in hysterics and though we all live miles away from
each other, I can still rely on them for laughs and love. Soph
bought us all a little cactus each and Karis said I should have
titled this drawing "Six Pricks," which would have been
accurate.

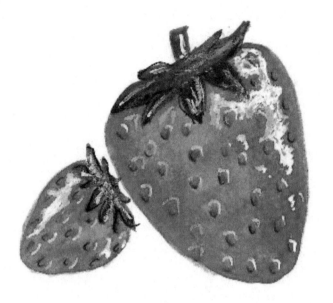

SWEET TASTE OF SUMMER.

It's so lovely to finally feel like summer is here and one of the best things is having strawberries that actually taste like they should. Milo thought he was being sneaky but we all noticed the chubby little hand reaching into the punnet.

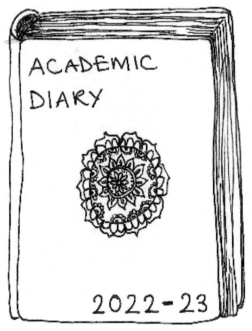

NEW BEGINNINGS.

Today, I officially accepted an offer to train as an Art
Psychotherapist at Roehampton starting in September. It's
exciting and nerve wrecking, all at the same time. Part of me
feels like I am tempting fate and by accepting, I am not going
to be in good enough health to be able to do it. However, as
Harry pointed out, I need to keep planning things into my life
and this is something I've been talking about for a long time
so now feels like as good a time as any.

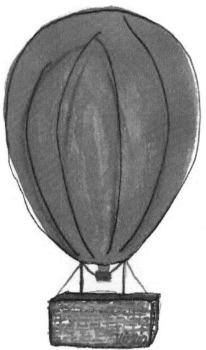

ADVENTURE AWAITS.

On our way home today, we saw people setting up a hot air balloon in a local field. Milo wanted to stay and watch but knowing it would be a while, I carried on home trying to convince him we'd see it go past our house. Sure enough during bath time, we saw the ⓐvirgin balloon drifting past and Milos eyes lit up. I've always wanted to go in one so I have decided I'm going to go ahead and arrange it because life is too short to simply 'want' to do something.

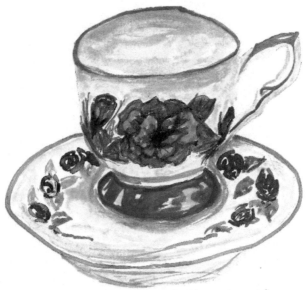

AFTERNOON TEA.

Today, I went to see my lovely friend Swifty for lunch. She made a tasty ceaser salad then for dessert served up some delicious home-made scones. She brought out these gorgeous tea cups and it felt very apt with it being the Queen's Jubilee. Hope everyone has a wonderful bank holiday weekend!

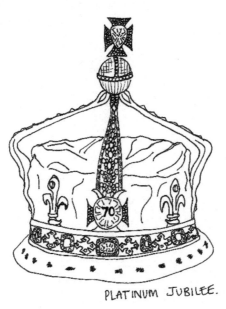

PLATINUM JUBILEE.

We took full advantage of the sunny bank holiday by spending the morning at the beach with Nana and Baba, followed by a BBQ with friends this afternoon. I realised while I was sitting there in the sunshine, drinking beer and chatting, that I didn't feel rubbish. I actually feel 'normal.' I mean, don't get me wrong, some side effects are out staying their welcome but on the whole, it's sooo much better. Hope everyone had a fabulous day in the sunshine!

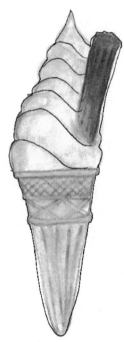

FESTIVITIES.

Busy day! Met with Lottie at Frensham Great pond for a dip before heading to Harting Festivities. We used to go all the time as a child so it was nice to be able to take Milo. We ticked off all the village fete musts; dog show, brass band, craft stalls, carousel, raffle, chips at the pub and finished with an ice cream. The sun was shining most of the day but of course, there was the obligatory shower. Happy Platty Joobs everyone!

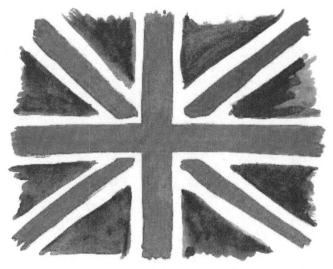

PROUD TO BE BRITISH.

I can't say I'm particularly patriotic but watching the Jubilee concert this evening I'm feeling pretty proud. Sure, some of it is questionable but on the whole, it's pretty damn enjoyable and a little ray of light amongst all the crap going on in the world right now.

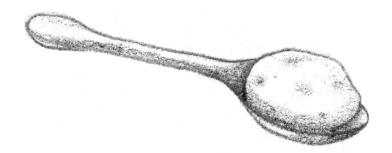

SPOON & ~~EGG~~ & POTATO RACE.

After a lovely walk with the Flints this morning, we had lunch at our favourite pub, the Noah's Ark, in Lurgashall. There was a little fete going on the green and once we'd finished eating, we wandered over. It was so quaint and there was a sweet old man running it. They announced an egg and spoon race and Harry took Milo to join in. He was handed his spoon and a potato (I guess they are cheaper than eggs) and took his place in the line-up, by far the smallest of the kids. They set off and Milo instantly dropped it so Harry, who is extremely competitive, bent to pick it up then held it onto Milos spoon while pushing him along. He crossed the finish line last but had the biggest grin on his face which absolutely made my day. To cap it off, there was a magic show which was actually really cute and Milo was enthralled. What a round off to a very wholesome weekend.

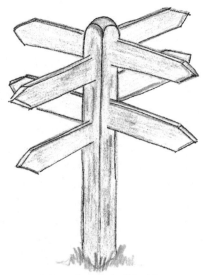

DECISION MAKING.

Since finishing chemo, I have felt lost, like I have been cast out and I'm floating around in space trying to grab hold of something. Having the surgery dates in has helped, but there are still so many questions and possible outcomes. Then to add to the mix, last week my doctor rings to tell me that they have changed the guidelines so I now qualify for genetic testing to see if I have a faulty gene. This has thrown everything up in the air and I'm now questioning earlier decisions. Another appointment today and more options will be presented. My brain is frazzled and I want to curl into a ball and ignore it. Luckily, I have a great support system and I know that I'll make the right choice for me in the end. Just part of the process.

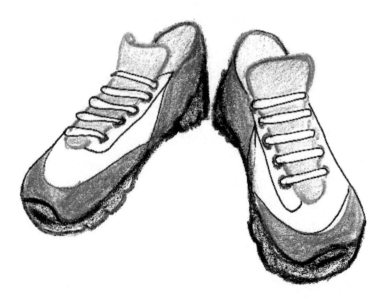

BACK ON MY FEET.

This morning, I went for my first run in over 6 months. I was in no way an avid (or very good) runner before my diagnosis but was able to go for a slow 5k if I wanted. The last few months, I have barely had the energy for day to day activities, never mind actual exercise. But as my energy seeps back, I am eager to get my fitness back and take back ownership of my body. Today's run was barely that, I walked on and off (mainly up the hills) but I did manage a few longer stretches and it felt good. Feels like I am clawing back some of what I have lost.

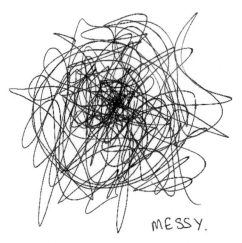

MESSY.

After a lovely morning of creating (painting and pottery) then lunch and a visit to an art gallery with Mum, I was feeling pretty relaxed and like myself. But as the evening arrived and I hadn't had a call from the doctor that I was expecting, I'm left feeling frustrated and confused. Still unsure about what to do about my surgery next week. Hopefully I will speak to someone tomorrow and get some clarity.

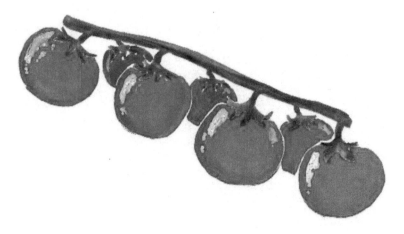

TOMATOES ON THE VINE.

This morning, Harry and I went for a long walk into the
village to buy some fruit and veg from the green grocers.
Sounds ridiculously quaint I know. Milo thought it was a 'help
yourself' situation and plucked a ripe tomato off the vine and
popped it into his mouth. Cheeky monkey. Luckily, the owner
was lovely and just smiled. This evening, I was surprised by
my gorgeous girlfriends for dinner at a wonderful Greek
restaurant. Feel so spoilt and loved.

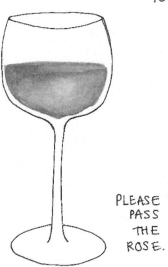

PLEASE
PASS
THE
ROSE.

Last night, I got to have dinner with some of my beautiful
girl friends (missed those that couldn't make it) and it was a
really wonderful evening of delicious food and rose. We met at
college fifteen years ago and no matter the distance and time
that comes between us, we can always get together and have
a laugh. Not only that, but when I was diagnosed, these girls
made sure I felt loved and supported by the way of parcels
and regular messages of love. They are all one in a million and
I'm so so grateful for them. So todays post is to say thank
you to my gals!

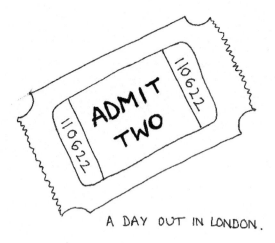

A DAY OUT IN LONDON.

As a special treat for my oldest pal, Ella, who is getting married in three weeks, I arranged a day of surprises in London including the Cartoon museum. Yes, we're cool kids. There was an immersive dining experience as well. We never fail to have a good time and actually the best thing about the day was walking through London Town nattering away.

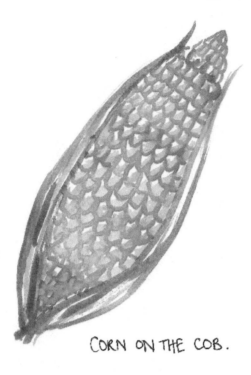

CORN ON THE COB.

Today was the perfect day of walks, sunshine and a BBQ with
wonderful friends. The corn on the cob was particularly
delicious. Hope everyone had a lovely weekend.

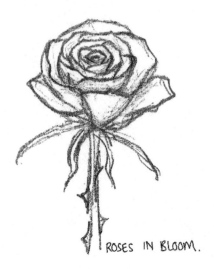

ROSES IN BLOOM.

Spent the afternoon in the garden with Mum and Milo admiring the flowers and tackling the weeds. Milo has developed a very mischievous streak recently. He disappeared for a while and when I called him back, he had red juice round his mouth and a small red berry in his hand. Before I could get close enough to see what it was, he ran off and when I followed him round the back of the shed, there was a whole crop of wild strawberries. Milo had already made a pretty large dent but we were able to pick the rest and hide them in the fridge.

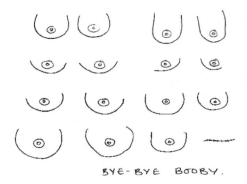

BYE-BYE BOOBY.

Breasts, boobs, tits or tattas, whatever you call them, they come in all shapes and sizes. Today I had an appointment with the surgeons who will be doing my surgery on Friday. It has been planned for a while and was going to be a fairly simple surgery to remove the sentinel lymph node (the first one to drain off the breast tissue) as well as a few others. They then get sent off to the lab to be tested for cancer cells; if it comes back positive they remove most of the rest but if they are negative, they can close me up. I had then planned to have the mastectomy and reconstruction two weeks later. However, after my oncologist expressed concern that it was too bigger delay, I freaked out. So we started exploring other options and the surgeon suggested I have the mastectomy this Friday as well. This sounded like the best option as I will have the cancer removed as soon as possible.

However, there is a caveat... my reconstruction is no longer urgent so I get put on a waiting list which is currently over a year. A year of feeling lopsided and incomplete. It felt like an impossible decision but after talking it over with my Mum and Harry, I realised the most important thing is to be cancer free. I'm sure I'll learn to live with it and eventually love it.

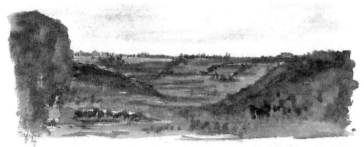

TEMPLE OF THE WINDS.

Today was spent in isolation. If you have Covid then you can't have surgery for seven weeks due to the complications that can arise. So I had a PCR yesterday and have another on Friday morning and channeling all my energy into hoping they come back negative so they can operate. Mum has taken Milo to reduce the risk so I spent the day by myself which was actually quite nice. This evening, once the temperature had dropped, I took moose out for a walk. I decided I fancied climbing up Blackdown, the big hill near our house. It felt amazing to have the energy to climb it, especially considering that only a couple of months ago I would have laughed at the suggestion. I didn't see another soul but had my mask with me just in case. It was over four miles in total and 235m ascent. The view at the top was phenomenal and added to the feeling of accomplishment.

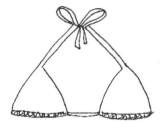

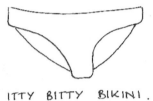

ITTY BITTY BIKINI.

Another day in isolation so I decided to take advantage of the sun and pop on my bikini for some sunbathing. It'll be a while before I can wear one like this and I've been told by a few people to take some photos of myself before surgery. So here I am, soaking up the rays.

ALL CLEAR.

After a long wait, I'm finally back on the ward. The surgery
went well and the test on the lymph nodes came back clear
which is a huge relief. They have sent them off for further
testing just to be sure. The surgeon was pleased with the
mastectomy but was concerned about swelling so kept me in
overnight but then the nurses were concerned about my blood
pressure so kept me in recovery for ages. Luckily, they bought
me a cup of sweet tea which helped my sore throat. Now time
to try and get some sleep.

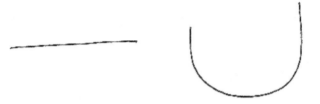

RECOVERY.

Back home this evening and all snuggled up on the sofa. Woke this morning feeling pretty sore but the nurses kept the painkillers flowing. The surgeon came in to check the wound and said that it was looking good so I could go home. I have a drain which has to stay in for a week to make sure the wound doesn't swell up. The breast cancer nurses gave me a little heart pillow to go under my arm which has been there all day. Thank you all for the support and messages of love, it really does make all the difference and means the world to me.

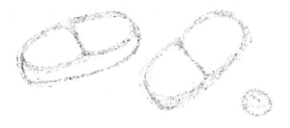

PAIN RELIEF.

Haven't got a lot of strength in my right arm at the moment so this little sketch is all I can muster. Every four hours, I get to take these three little pills (Codine and paracetamol) which keep the worst of the pain at bay. Though a side effect is I feel very woozy and out of it. The other form of pain relief is cuddles with my little man as well as visits from friends and family which make the world of difference.

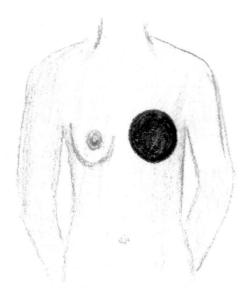

INCOMPLETE .

Starting to feel a little more like myself today and a little less sore. The general anaesthetic is finally wearing off and I'm feeling less woozy. This evening, I managed to have a little bath and look at the reflection staring back at me. It's still a shock but each time I get a little more used to seeing the empty space where part of me used to be. I know it's not forever but certainly need to come to accept it until I have reconstruction.

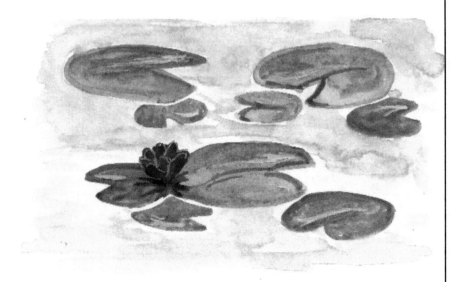

LILY PADS ON THE POND.

Woke today with a little more strength and a little less pain. The doctor called to ask about my drain and how much has come out (sorry bit gross). Basically, he explained that as the last two days there had been less than 50ml, I could have it removed. Harry drove me up to the hospital so that the doctor could pull it out which made me feel really faint Anyhoo, nice not to carry it around anymore and I spent the afternoon sitting in the garden next to the little pond.

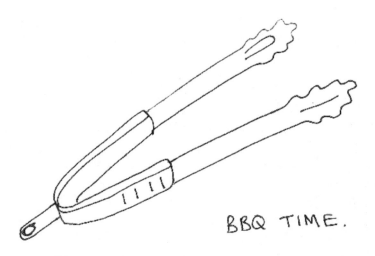

BBQ TIME.

Harry took the week off work to look after me (and Milo) as I am unable to do normal things like lifting while I recover from surgery. It's actually been really lovely the last couple of days as I've been able to do a bit more and enjoy the sunshine with Harry while Milo is at nursery. It's felt a bit like being on holiday with the gorgeous weather, lots of BBQs and endless card games. I didn't do a Father's Day post because I was so out of it, but I do have to say how amazing Harry is at being a Dad and I'm so unbelievably grateful for him. The relationship he has with Milo is adorable and I love watching them play together.

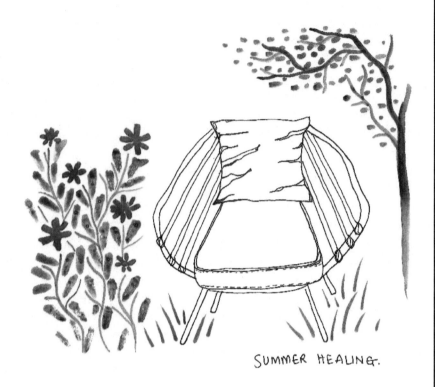

SUMMER HEALING.

After an appointment with the nurse to get my dressings changed, we took Milo for lunch to the café, which is one of our favourites. We always joke whenever we go in there, we end up coming out having bought something and sure enough... as we were leaving I spotted these two gorgeous chairs for the garden which were on clearance. I decided to treat myself and got them to be able to relax in our beautiful garden.

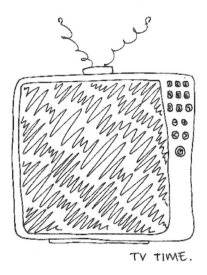

TV TIME.

After a busy afternoon yesterday, I felt wiped and achey this morning. I spent most of the morning watching TV as I couldn't muster the energy or motivation to do much else. This is the reality of recovery... there are ups and downs/ good days and bad days. It's also give and take... I have to realise if I want to do a lot then I need to make time for rest too. I guess that applies to everyone really, a quiet day is not a wasted day but a valuable day. Also my sister in law gave me The Hills on DVD so I borrowed my parents DVD player and am working through the seasons. It's so nostalgic and making me miss the 'good ol'days' when technology was so simple.

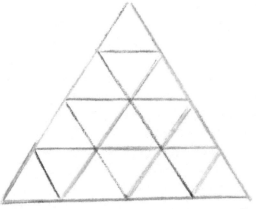

HOW MANY TRIANGLES?

Every year, Harry and I watch Glastonbury on the TV and spend most of the time wishing we were there. We've never been able to go due to me being a teacher and Harry having a silly job where he can't get time off. However, we have decided that we are going to put it off no longer and going to do what we can to get there for next year so we can see pyramid stage for ourselves. Also here's a little riddle for you to try, how many triangles can you see in this pyramid?

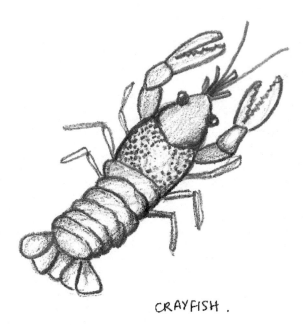

CRAYFISH .

Feeling pretty sore now as the numbing injection they gave me during the surgery has worn off so I can feel the wound more keenly. However, I had some wonderful friends and sunshine to distract me today. We went to Frensham Ponds and the others all went for a dip while I watched from the beach. As they were heading into the water, a man came out carrying a bucket with a crayfish floating in it. I had no idea you could get them in the lake so was amazed but also slightly relieved I had an excuse for not being able to go in, as the thought of them scuttling round my feet creeped me out a little! Hope everyone had a wonderful weekend.

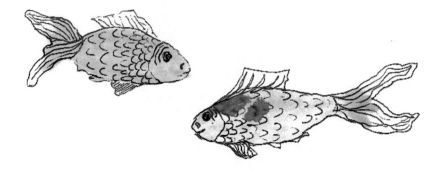

GO FISH.

Today, Grandma and I took Milo to the Garden Centre to buy some more fish for our pond. We chose 2 pink ones and decided to name them Pinky and Perky. Milo was very excited to pop them into our pond then we realised we should probably name the other three which Milo insisted last summer should all be called 'fish'. He's a little more imaginative now so we have satsuma, buttercup and rainbow. The family is complete.

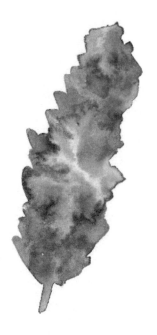

WATERCOLOUR FEATHER

Another day and a little bit stronger and more myself. The wound hurts a lot less now and I've got most of the movement back in my arm... just have to be careful with lifting. Treated myself to a pedicure as I had a gift voucher from someone lovely, and they had the most beautiful wallpaper with feathers. While I was chatting to the technician I told her that my nails had fallen apart since having chemo. It came out of my mouth easily and I continued to chat about my diagnosis without getting emotional. However, at one point I did catch myself and it still feels so surreal. It probably hasn't sunk in yet and I imagine won't for sometime....

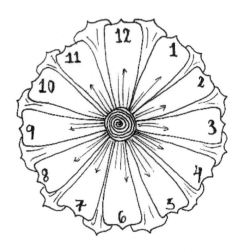

TIME.

I've been thinking a lot recently about time, then with the death of the absolute babe that is Dame Deborah James at only 41 years old, I am reminded again that sometimes there is simply not enough. In the last 7 months, my time, a little like for everyone during Covid, has been warped. Some days stretch on forever while other pass on a blink of an eye. Like many others going through treatment, I have been robbed of many things but the bizarre thing is I feel like I have been gifted time. I have spent way more time with Milo, Harry, my Mum and friends and family than I would have done if I was working and living a 'normal' life. Though a lot of this may have been me slumped on the sofa while people work hard to chat with me or slow walks, I have treasured the feeling of being loved.

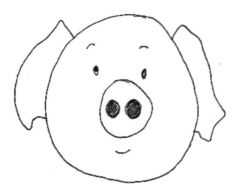

PIGGY.

Today we drove down to Devon for the wedding of my oldest and most loveliest friend, Ella. It's not till Saturday but we wanted to come and help set up. It's on the families farm and I used the fact there would be pigs as a way to get Milo to behave on the journey down. Unfortunately, the pigs turned out to be massive and pretty loud with their grunts which had Milo terrified. This evening, we had a dinner for Ella with a few friends and everyone wore a pig snout because when Ella was younger she had a strange obsession with pigs and collected them in all forms. It was such a lovely evening and when I got back I completely forgot, I hadn't done my drawing for today... so here it is, a little Piggy.

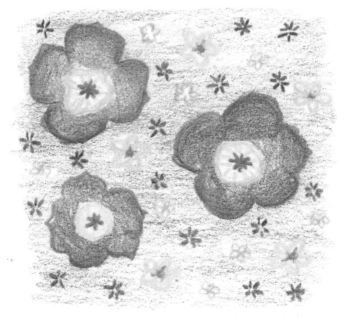

FLOWER POWER.

A day of wedding prep today which involved putting out vintage beer mats, hanging disco balls and draping awesome 70s themed fabrics that Ella found in a thrift shop. The overall effect is awesome and I'm so excited for tomorrow! Also we got to meet the piglets today which was much more successful as Milo loved their little squeals.

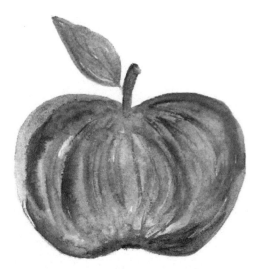

THE APPLE OF MY EYE.

Ella's wedding day. I have known this girl since we were two years old and I can honestly say that she is the most reliable, loyal, hilarious and lovely person. I am so grateful for her everyday. She just gifted me some amazing Somerset cider flavoured gin from Still Sisters Distillery in Frome where she lives. Such a thoughtful gift and so apt as she really is 'the apple of my eye' Today is going to be AMAZING and I am so excited for her to be completely showered in love.

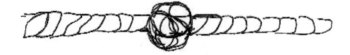

TUG OF WAR.

One of the pinnacle moments of the wedding yesterday was the tug of war between the 2 families. It was unbelievably competitive and there were a lot of people getting knocked down and covered in grass stains. Milo was desperate to get involved! However, it was all smiles in the end and everyone earned themselves a drink. I have felt in a tug of war with my body today. It feels battered and bruised despite the fact I didn't even take part. Just doing 'normal' activities seems to completely knock me out. TOTALLY worth it though and memories to cherish forever. Most of them are from the dance floor and in particular when Milo was on Harry's shoulders and they played 'sister sledge-we are family' which we sing with Milo all the time.

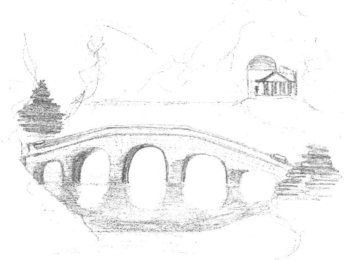

STOURHEAD GARDENS.

Drove back from Devon today and stopped off at Stourhead
for some lunch. It was a stunning place and the sun was
shining so it was a lovely way to round off an incredible
weekend. Finally home and back on the sofa this evening feeling
exhausted but so content. So so lucky to not only have my
cheeky little boy but also my beautiful friends and family.

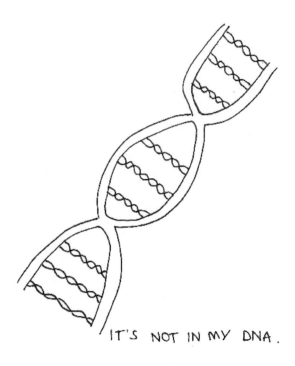

IT'S NOT IN MY DNA.

Today, I had the great news from my genetics test that I do not have a faulty gene which increases the risk of getting cancer. However, this does mean that the fact that I did develop cancer at 31 is just damn unlucky! But hey ho, it's still reason to celebrate!

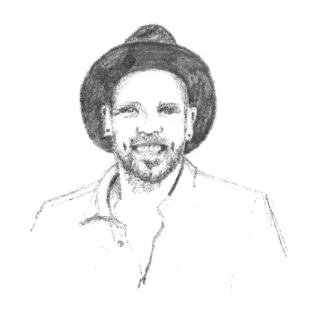

MY HARRY.

Today is Harry's birthday so we're celebrating with a curry from one of our favourites which we have only just found out delivers here so we're very excited! Harry and I met at university in freshers week over 11 years ago and what drew me to him was his cheeky grin and dimples. We became inseparable fairly quickly and he's been my person ever since. Though we have our moments and we are no way perfect, life without him would be a lot less fun. So here's to my best friend, my rock, my Harry.

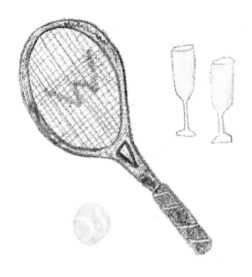

WATCHING THE TENNIS.

Last night, Milo was super sick and none of us got much sleep, including the washing machine which has done at least 5 loads in the last 24 hours. That meant today was a wipe out, despite the fact Milo perked up after he kept breakfast down, and I was totally exhausted so spent some time on the sofa watching Tennis. In previous years, I've gone after work with my good friend Lottie and we've shared a bottle of Prosecco while sitting on the hill watching on the big screen. It's sad not to attend this year but still fun to watch from afar!

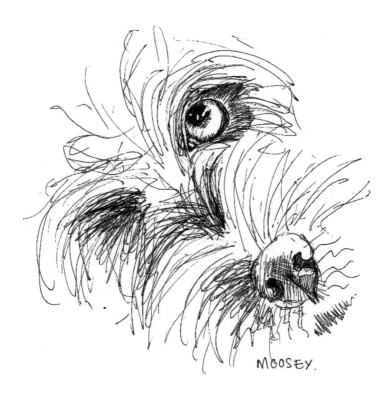

MOOSEY.

A beautiful day of sunshine. Took Milo to get his haircut today and he's looking so grown up, it scares me! While he napped, I chilled in the garden with moose, my little pal.

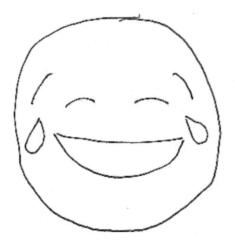

LAUGHING OUT LOUD.

Tonight, we went to a local comedy night with our nearest and dearest. Zoe Lyons was absolutely hilarious and I certainly appreciated all her bald jokes!!

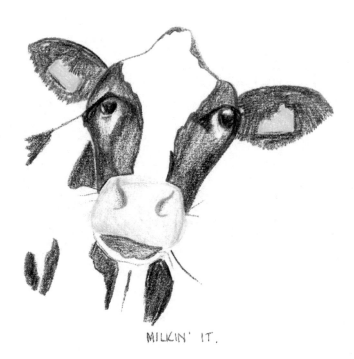

MILKIN' IT.

Today, we went for lunch for Harry's birthday at the Coppa club in Sonning. He's reeeeally milking it this year. Afterwards, we walked along the river and passed some very curious cows. Harry even took a little dip in the cool water and we persuaded Milo to join him along with his cousins which was so magical to watch. What a beautiful weekend!

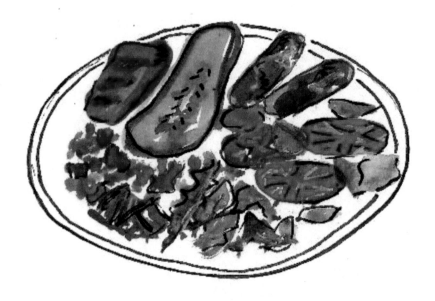

A COLOURFUL PLATE.

This evening, my cousin arrived from California with his daughter and boyfriend so we had a BBQ in our garden. It's the first evening that we've managed to eat outside and actually not feel cold which was amazing and so good to catch up with my overseas family.

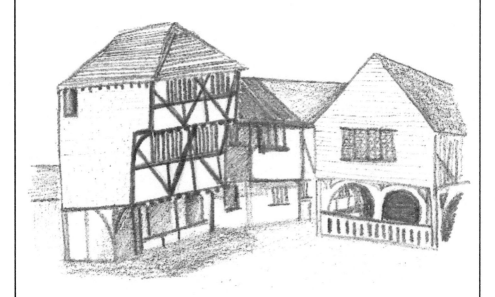

WEALD & DOWNLAND OPEN AIR MUSEUM .

Today, we took my cousin and family to Weald & Downland open air museum in Singleton. I used to go there a lot when I was younger, so it was very nostalgic but also so fun to see Milo running round the houses which are actual houses from various periods in history.

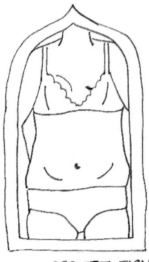

REFLECT-TION

Lately, I have been unbelievably bloated, whether it's a lasting effect of the chemo, the menopause or my IBS flaring up. I look like I did when I was pregnant with Milo. It's hard not to feel fed up when I see it and I know that most women experience fairly regularly but some much worse than the others. It's infuriating as you wake up okay, eat barely anything then bloat as if you've eaten a full Christmas dinner. I thought it was alcohol so I have stopped drinking but that hasn't helped. I thought maybe dairy made it worse so haven't had any but no change. Thinking I should get in touch with a nutritionist to work something out so if anyone has a good one, please let me know.

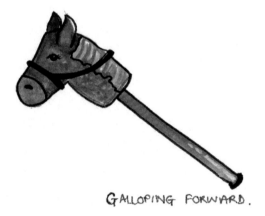

GALLOPING FORWARD.

Today, we found a couple of little ride along horses in the
charity shop and Milo absolutely loved playing with them so we
bought them home. He spent all day clip clopping around the
house which was adorable then when his buddy came over,
they were galloping around the garden. I am still awaiting my
results from the surgery and though, I am trying desperately
to look forward and be positive, I can't help glancing behind me
as if something terrible is about to happen. The longer I have
to wait, the more agonising it becomes. I am channeling all my
energy into a good result

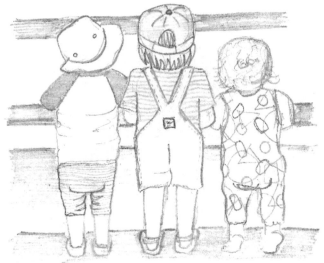

BEST OF FRIENDS.

Today, we went to Fishers farm with my best friends and their little ones. Watching the three of them together brings me so much joy and absolutely melts my heart. Love them all so much.

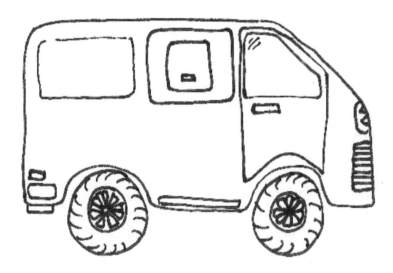

RHINO THE VAN

Woke up this morning to the crap news that someone nicked Harry's van last night while it was parked outside a friend's house in Bristol. So sad as we have so many amazing memories in that van including camping trips and the photo booth for our wedding! Gutted. However, spent the day at a school friend's wedding which has been an amazing reunion and so good catching up with people I haven't seen in over ten years!

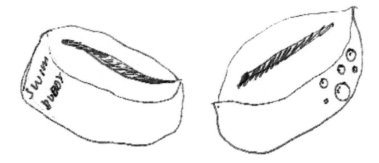

SWIMMING LESSONS.

So this morning, we took Milo to my parent's neighbour's pool for a swim. He is starting to gain confidence in the water and learning the movements which is making me super proud. This afternoon, we went for a BBQ at our neighbours house which was so wonderful watching Milo run around with his friends.

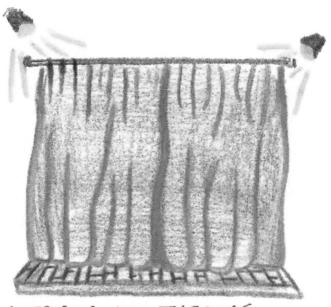

A TRIP TO THE THEATRE.

This evening, Mum took me to the Chichester theatre to see 'Crazy for You' which was amazing. The actors were all incredible and really admired them for carrying on in this heat. If you're local and love a musical, I definitely recommend.

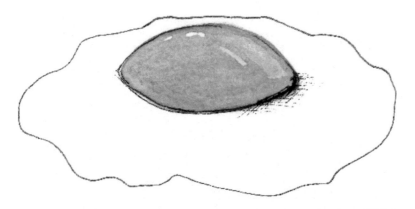

HOT ENOUGH TO FRY AN EGG

Sheeeeesh, today was hot, as my very good friend Rory said, "hot enough to fry an egg." Here in the UK, we don't cope well in the heat and spend most of the day using different words to describe the temperature "a scorcher/redders/stifling etc" and finding ways to cool down. My favourite is sitting with my feet in a bucket. Having children in this heat really makes you step up your game and just desperately trying to keep their sweaty bodies at arms length! If this weather doesn't wake us all up to Climate change, I'm not sure what will.

———————

NEGATIVE.

Today, I finally had a meeting with the oncologist about my results. It was good news. Great news, in fact. The lab has found that after examining the breast tissue that they removed, there were no active cancer cells. Only scar tissue. What this means is that the chemo completely killed the cells and wiped out the cancer.

Negative is not a word we usually want to hear but in this case, it is exactly what I have been day dreaming about for the last eight months since my diagnosis. When he told us, I actually burst out crying.

A mix of relief and disbelief. When you've had terrible news, you kinda come to expect it. It still hasn't sunk in and probably won't for a while.

It was certainly nice to be able to call my family and share good news. But I did it. I actually kicked cancers butt. The journey is far from over as I have to be on preventative drugs for a few years, yet but for now I can finally breath again.

Thank you to all those of you who have supported me through this. I simply could not have done it without you. Also a big shout out to the NHS for literally saving my life and taking such good care of me.

I may feel 20 years older, have one boob left and a new hairstyle amongst other things, but I am. here. And I am grateful beyond belief.

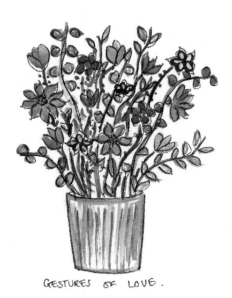

GESTURES OF LOVE.

I have spent the last day feeling a huge sense of relief as well as being overwhelmingly grateful. The messages of love from people I have known forever, a short time, those I haven't seen for far too long and lots of whom I have never met but have connected with on this journey, have been wonderful. I have received countless cards, gifts, and bouquets of flowers which have the meant the absolute world to me. It really does take a village to beat something like this and I am so incredibly lucky to be surrounded by such loving and generous people. All that love and positive vibes that were sent over the last few months kept me strong, so thank you. All of you.

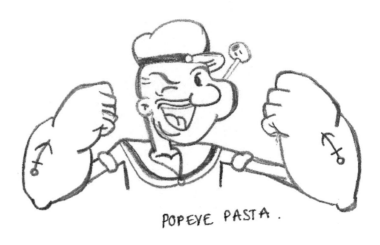

POPEYE PASTA .

Today, I made Popeye pasta, a recipe a friend gave me which is basically blitzed spinach with cream cheese and a little lemon. Milo loved it, probably because it was bright green but it also tasted delicious. I decided to show him a picture of Popeye for reference and he was totally perplexed. To be honest, I can see why, how bizarre is this cartoon? I mean he has ridiculously big forearms and non-existent upper arms?! Anyhoo, I am slightly jealous that all he has to do is down a can of spinach and he's super strong... I wish getting my strength back was that easy! Slow and steady Claire, slow and steady.

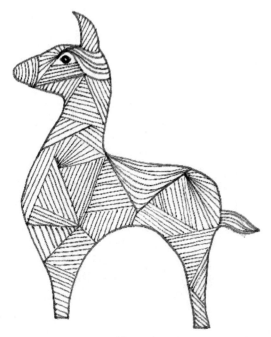

NO PROB-LLAMA

My gorgeous sister in law, Kathryn, has always loved a play on word so when I saw a mug with this on it, I couldn't resist. Also, it's my new mantra, just taking it easy.

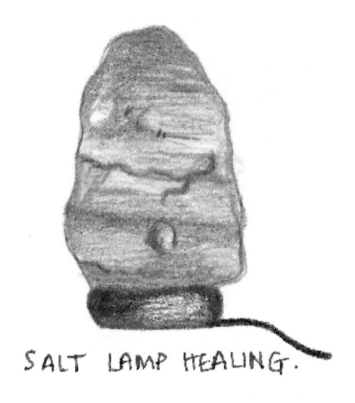

SALT LAMP HEALING.

After a wonderful evening with pals last night, my beautiful
friends Anna and Em gifted me a salt lamp. I have always
wanted one, as in theory, they clean the air and can boost your
mood. Again I am so touched by the generosity of my loved
ones. Today, we spent the day with my cousins and while we
sat in the sunshine; eating delicious food, drinking cold beer and
watching the kids jumping into the pool, it felt so damn good
to be alive.

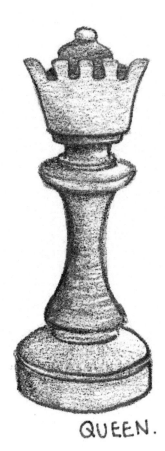

QUEEN.

I just beat Harry in Chess and it feels goood. We got into it after watching the Queens Gambit during lock down. My Pappie bought me a chess board last year as Harry already had the pieces and it's beautiful.

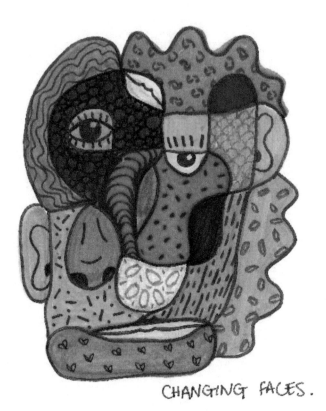

CHANGING FACES.

As a part of trying to progress into my creative career, while not letting go of teaching, I have finally gotten round to setting up an Etsy shop. Let's see how it goes.

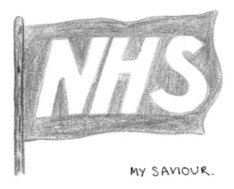

MY SAVIOUR.

Today, it was back to hospital for no#6/18 of my injection. As I followed the familiar route to the Chemo ward, I could feel my heart rate rising (the stairs probably didn't help...!) and I started to feel nauseous. The sound of the infusion machine beeping sent me into a bit of a frenzy and as I walked past the wards and glanced in to see the patients receiving their chemo, I felt like I was heading toward a full on panic attack. It's incredible how simple sights and sounds can cause such a strong physiological response. However, it was soon okay as I entered the TYA ward and was greeted by the familiar smiling faces of the nurses. The injection I got was a drug known as Herceptin, which was only invented about 20 years ago. It is used in HER2 positive breast cancer and has completely changed the prognosis. I am so incredibly grateful for the NHS and all the organisations that research these incredible medicines. Without them, I'd be facing a much bigger mountain. Thank goodness for scientists

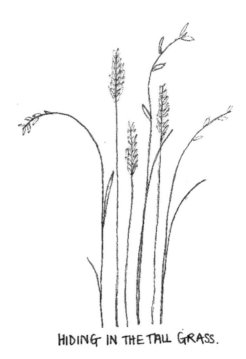

HIDING IN THE TALL GRASS.

This evening, Milo and I took Moose for a walk in the evening
sunshine. We played hide and seek in the long grass which Milo
found hilarious. On a side note, I feel like I am more
camouflaged when I go out and about now that my hair is at
a normal length. I don't feel like people do a double take at me
wearing a beanie/headscarf or bald. Feel like I am
returning/evolving.

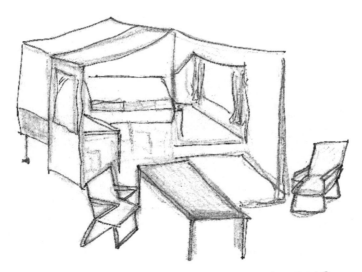

OLD SCHOOL CAMPING.

We're away camping in Dorset with my family this weekend and my brother has his Trailer tent which is identical to the one we had when we were younger. It's so nostalgic and magical to reminisce on memories while creating new ones. I actually managed to run around playing football earlier which felt amazing. The boys are currently having their bath time in the tubs, the sun is setting and the beer is cold. Life is so, so good.

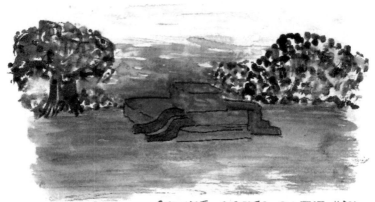

BEDTIME STORIES ON THE HAY.

We spent an amazing day at Studland Bay beach, one of our favourites down in Dorset. Last time we were on that beach, it was Easter and I had just had a round of chemo. I remember sitting on the beach wrapped in a blanket, feeling like absolute crap. Today was a complete contrast; I went swimming, out on the SUP and played with Milo in the sand. It really highlights to me just how shit I felt at the time and how much more normal I am now. After a quick pint at the Scott's Arms on the way home and a much needed shower, the children on the campsite all started heading towards the hay bales set up in the middle. The farmer arrived with her dogs to tell a bed time story. The children sat on the grass, listening intently as the sun set behind us. It was definitely one of those memories I never want to lose.

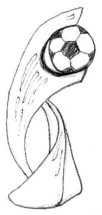

IT's HOME.

Amazing weekend finished in the most incredible way - watching the lionesses bring it home. I'm not hugely into football but watching the team play this championship has been inspirational. What a bladdy awesome group of athletes who not only worked damn hard but had a lot of fun. Congratulations Lionesses.

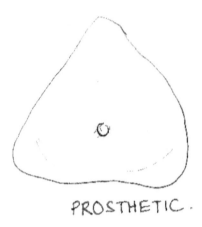

PROSTHETIC.

Today, I had a fitting for my breast prosthetic. I had taken a photo of my mastectomy scar so I could share it with this post but as I selected it, I suddenly choked. My reasons for doing it were to normalise mastectomy scars and to desensitise for those who are heading that way, just like other women did for me. However, suddenly, I felt an overwhelming sense of vulnerability. In the past 9 months, I have been poked, prodded and examined by multiple people and no longer care about medical people seeing my torso. I have shown my scar to my close people and feel no shame, only pride. (Thank you to Dr Pooja at Royal Surrey for doing such a wonderful job.) I may change my mind and want to show you all but for now, it's a part of me that I get to keep private.

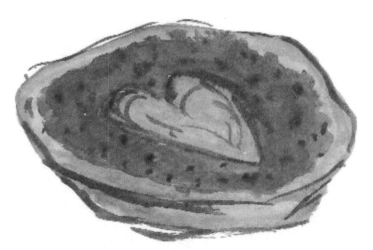

(NOT) QUEEN OF TARTS .

Today, I had a massage at the Fountain Centre which was great, all the Kim, the masseuse, was amazing and gave me loads of good advice for recovery. This afternoon, I made jam tarts with Milo. He was in charge of spooning the jam onto the pastry and it was only half way through that I noticed in between each spoonful into a tart, was a spoonful into his mouth. They turned out okay but I'm definitely not a baker.

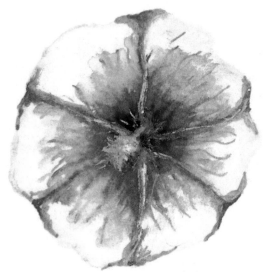

HIBISCUS.

Visited Wisley Gardens today with a lovely friend and was blown away by the beautiful blooms. It was so nice to wander slowly through the flowers rather than when I'm with Milo and we march straight to the playground, though it is a lot of fun.

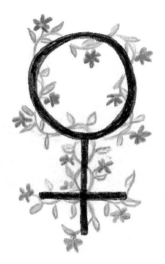

I AM WOMAN.

Menopause. Whether it's early, medically induced or when you were expecting it, it's a bugger. It's also not talked about enough despite affecting half the population. The symptoms sound innocent enough; hot flushes, night sweats, confusion, memory loss but in reality, they are horrible. They vary in severity from woman to woman but on the whole it is unpleasant. One of the worst, that I experienced this morning, is rage. It comes from nowhere and is hard to control. Some reading this may think that it's a matter of mind over matter but it's so much more than that. It feels like it is bubbling up inside and I had to work so hard to not to snap at Milo for the simplest of things. Frustrating. Anyway, to summarise, menopause is not talked about enough and if you're unsure of what it is/what it does... please feel free to go read up.

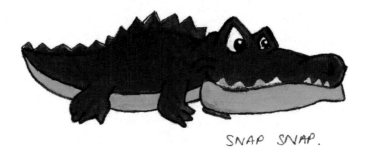

SNAP SNAP.

Today was a busy one that started at Durleigh Marsh Farm with some fruit picking. When Milo realised he could pop the blueberries into his mouth rather than the punnet, there was no stopping him. After, we went back to my Mums and I snuck out for a run. Then it was next door for a delicious swim, after which Milo refused to take off his crocodile towel and specifically said, "no pants but shoes on please Mummy." Finally, we took the dogs out for an evening walk and ended up discovering some juicy blackberries. The idea of a day this jam packed and snappy a couple months ago would have been ridiculous so it's crazy to me that I managed it. I know to most, this sounds so normal but to me it's getting my life back.

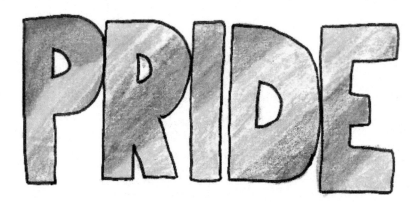

Brighton Pride today for the gorgeous Frankie's hen. The most magical, kind and loving crowd of people. Oh and Christina Aguilara is performing!!

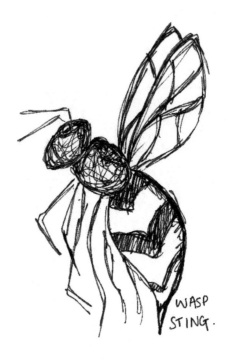

WASP STING.

Today, as I was walking into the house, a wasp flew under my little toe and stung me. The shock traveled through my body and I shouted "fucker" while grabbing at my foot. It throbbed for a while then started to fade. It made me think about how earlier, when I was making lunch, there was an advert for MacMillan on the radio and the girl was saying "when my Mum was diagnosed with cancer…" The physical response was the same as the sting. It traveled through my body and my heart did a back flip. It passed but for a short moment, I felt paralysed. I know it will soften as time moves on but at the moment, I think I am still in total shock and sometimes unsure that the last 8 months even happened.

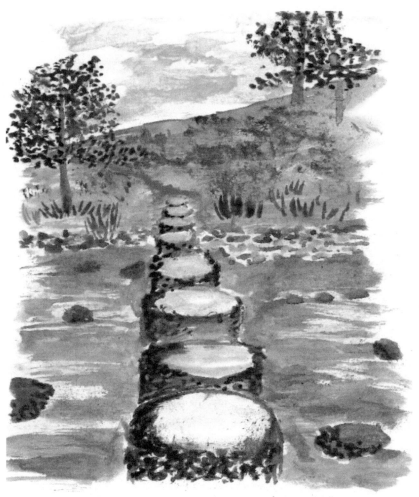

STEPPING STONES.

Today, Mum, Milo and I drove the long journey to Lancashire to stay in my Auntie Joan's cottage. We had an unbearable shock this time last year when we found out she had cancer and it had travelled to her brain. It was devastating news as she really was the kindest, most generous and loving person ever. We had a few weeks where we could visit her and I got to take Milo to meet her, as due to bloody COVID, we hadn't had a chance. We all miss her terribly and the end of this month will mark a year without her. I've thought of her lots but especially in the last few months. She would have been an incredible support through this and been there for my Mum but on the other hand, it is one person I was able to spare from the pain. Auntie Joan was always a huge fan of my art work and had a piece hanging in the living room here in the cottage, so I know she would be proud that I am using my creativity as a way of getting through. I feel like she is with me all the time, but particularly today when we visited the stepping stones near her house. It really felt like we were connected to her and I know she is so happy we are here. One of the poems that was read at her funeral finished with a line which was perfect for her....

"Open your eyes. Smile. Love and go on."

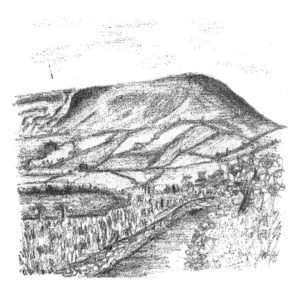

PENDLE HILL.

After Auntie Joan's cremation last September, we walked up Pendle Hill to scatter her ashes. It was her favourite place, after my Mums family grew up round here and Joan returned to bring up her sons in a nearby village. The hill can be seen from many points and is breathtaking at every angle. Any new addition to the family would be marched up there. Joan was the most gentle person I knew but when it came to walking, she literally did not hang about. It's a pretty steep climb and saying goodbye to her on top was hard but now we get to look at that beautiful hill and know she is happy up there, admiring the incredible view. Also, a little fact about the name - 'Pen' means hill and 'dle' also means hill so quite literally it's "Hillhill hill"

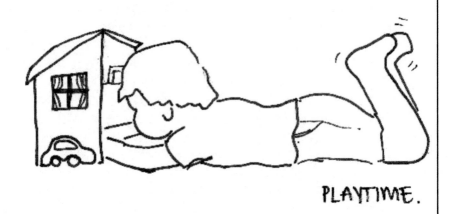

PLAYTIME.

Today, we visited some of my Mums extended family and they had got out a box of toys, most of which was probably older than me but of course that didn't stop Milo from diving in. He spent most of the time we were there, sprawled on the floor, playing with the little house. My Mum's cousin remarked on what a well behaved and polite little boy he was. When you spend 90% of the time with your toddler, you tend to remember the times they misbehave or have a tantrum so to hear how wonderful he really is, was a reminder to me of how lucky I am. This little boy is my absolute world and has coped with the last year so well. And to be fair, I've had waaaay more tantrums than him anyway.

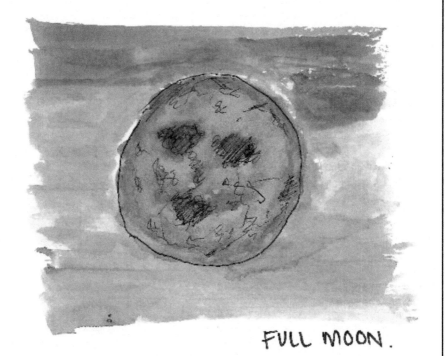

FULL MOON.

Finally home after driving over 280 miles. Was pretty exhausted by the end but the incredible full moon kept me going.

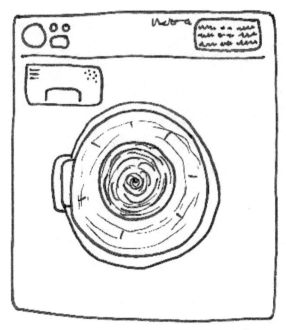

WASHING.

Whenever you go away, the day after you arrive home involves a silly amount of washing, no matter how long you were away for?! Also this is how I picture my brain at the moment, the thoughts and things I have to try and remember are constantly spinning around out of control. I catch a glimpse of something I wanted to tell someone, but it's gone the minute I open my mouth. I was warned about 'chemo brain' and thought it would start to improve once I was off treatment but it's taking its sweeeet time.

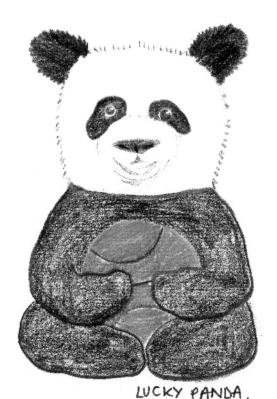

LUCKY PANDA.

A few years ago, I joined a basketball team, the Putney
Pandas, and got my own jersey with no. 18. I wasn't
particularly good but in my last game with them, I scored a
couple of lay ups and we won the game. Tonight when I was
looking for a t-shirt for my run, I pulled out my panda jersey
and set off. For the first time since I started running again a
few weeks ago, I actually felt really good and when I got to
the half way point, decided to take it a little further and
managed to do just over 6km. Clearly, this is my lucky shirt.

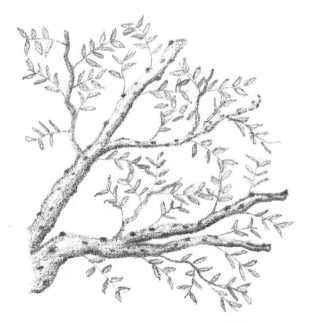

EUCALYPTUS .

We were supposed to see some very lovey friends this weekend but after a rather hectic and stressful time lately, we decided to cancel and have a weekend at home. It's been so nice just being the three of us and taking some time in our beautiful garden under the eucalyptus tree.

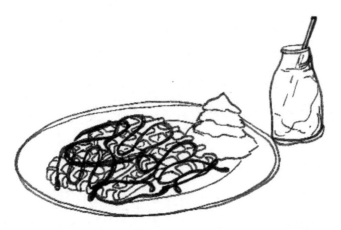

WAFFLES & MILKSHAKE.

This morning, I took Milo to get waffles and a milkshake at the lovely Fitzcanes. They were unbelievably good and Milo couldn't quite believe his luck that I was sharing with him. When I showed Harry the photo of them, he said, "Blimey, what was the special occasion?!" Life. Life is a bloody special occasion.

CUPCAKES.

After a quiet day of working on some art projects, I went to pick up Milo from nursery and we took Moosey for a walk along the river. He did really well despite the fact he was exhausted so we decided to go home and make cupcakes. We needed butter so I put Milo on my back for the walk up the high street to the shop. He said sweetly in my ear, "thank you for the piggy back Mummy." I almost burst into tears. Not being able to be the Mum I wanted to be for the first half of this year was the hardest thing so I'm so grateful my strength is returning. Oh and the cupcakes are pretty good if I don't say so myself.

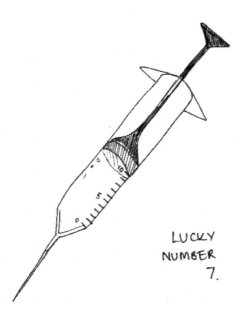

LUCKY
NUMBER
7.

Today, it was back up to the hospital and the TYAC ward for my 7th shot of Herceptin. Sam was there who was one of the first nurses I spoke to back in January after my first round of chemo. Despite being rushed off her feet, she came and sat with me and asked for my update. For some reason as I was telling her the good news, I broke down and she instantly wrapped me up in a hug. She totally understood why I was emotional and was so incredibly supportive. I could not be more grateful for the TYA nurses that have looked after me over the last year, they are absolute superheroes.

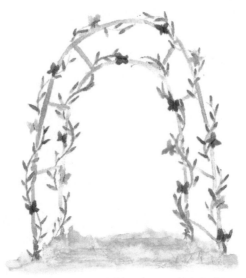

HAPPY ANNIVERSARY.

On this day, four years ago, Harry and I stood in front of our favourite people and said our vows. It really was the most magical day and the best bit about it was that I got to marry my best friend. Our first years of marriage have certainly thrown us some tests, but we are stronger than ever and I am so unbelievably grateful for Harry Team.

TO DO

- *(illegible)* — ple!!
- *(illegible)*
- *(illegible)* X.
- *(illegible)* !
- *(illegible)*
- *(illegible)* → our
- *(illegible)*
- *(illegible)*

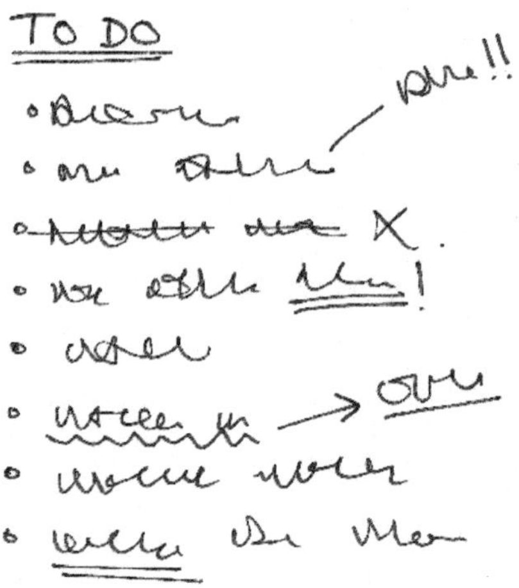

LISTS.

Today revolved around getting ready for our holiday which meant walking round the house, noticing things and adding them to the list. I don't know if it's because of having just gone through chemo/cancer or COVID but going out of the country this time feels so much more stressful. We haven't been away for 2 1/2 years and so are both very excited but also nervous. Feel like there are so many things that could go wrong?! Seems ironic that this time 4 years ago, Harry and I were off on our honeymoon with not a care in the world, still on cloud 9 from the wedding. Hopefully, it all goes smoothly.

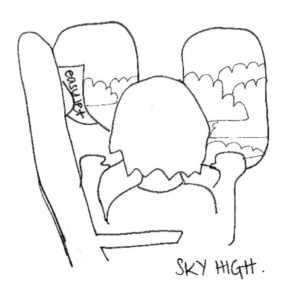

SKY HIGH.

After a LONG day of travelling, we made it. Milo LOVED the aeroplane and just couldn't get over that we were above the clouds. The queue for passport security took over 45 mins and he was an absolute angel. So proud of him. After a long drive up winding roads, we arrived at our beautiful chalet and our holiday has begun. Cheers everyone!

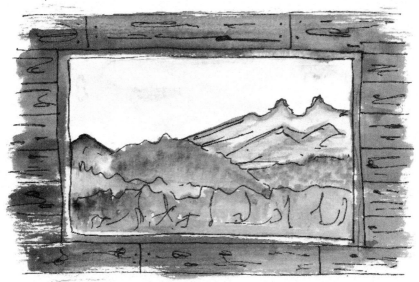

A VIEW WORTH FRAMING.

The mountain that this window frames is called "Roc D'Enfer" which means "Hell rock" but I can confirm this place is far from hell. Complete and utter heaven.

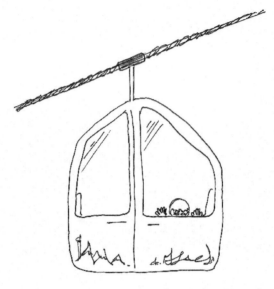

BUBBLES.

Today, we took Milo up the bubble lift. He's been talking about it since we arrived so was very excited. I don't think he anticipated how high up and bumpy the ride was but enjoyed it none the less and the view from the top was completely worth it.

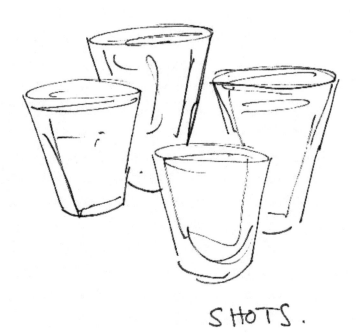

SHOTS.

The Nannas arrived yesterday so we went out this evening to eat and celebrate. It's the first time we've been out in a while so there were many drinks and a few shots... the worst being the 'Suze' that Harry ordered. Sooo good to have fun with good friends.

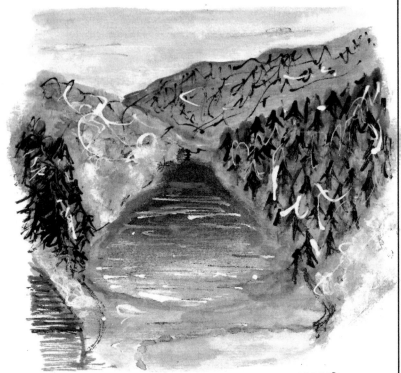

LAC DE MONTRIOND.

Today, we were up early (despite the hangover) to celebrate my god daughter Olive's 1st Birthday. After a croissant breakfast, we headed out and took another bubble up the mountain for some more phenomenal views. The afternoon was spent at the lake, swimming and playing in the sand. I never want to leave this place!

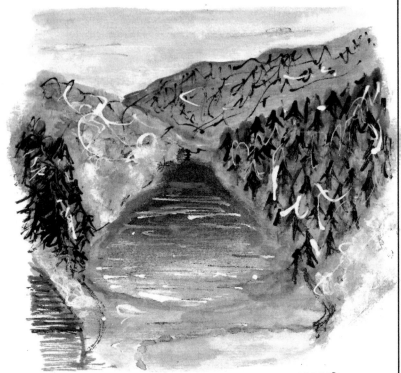

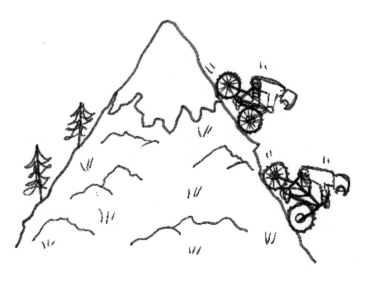

MOUNTAIN BIKING.

Today, Harry and Nick spent the day on the mountain getting the lift up then hurtling down at 60 kmh. Harry took a pretty nasty fall which I'm glad I wasn't there to see! In contrast, we had a lovely day pottering around town and sitting by the pool.

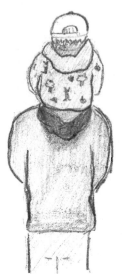

FEELING INSPIRED.

Today, we went over the Les Gets to watch the Mountain Bike World Championships. Milo was in absolute awe and sat on Harry's shoulders to watch the short track where they tore around a course of up and downhill and over massive rocks. It was really impressive and, despite the rain, we enjoyed the day.

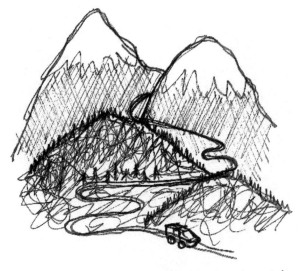

WINDING DOWN.

This morning, we packed up and made our way down the mountain. The road was pretty bendy and hairy at times but the views made it worth it. We've had an incredible week in the Alps but are looking forward to the second half of our holiday on the coast which will be much slower and we can finally relax. After 8 hours of driving already, we are just over an hour away and ready for bed.

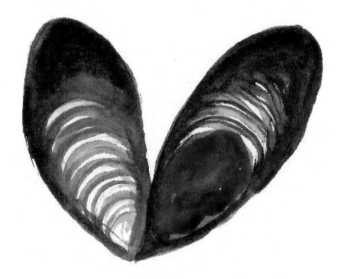

MOULES - FRITES

Today, we started the second part of our holiday by visiting the market in the local town and having a croissant and coffee. Then we had a splash in the pool before heading down to the beach for the late afternoon sun. We ended the day at dinner and Harry and I shared Mussels and sardines, which were delicious. Milo spent the time racing around with the other children laughing his head off. Felt like total heaven.

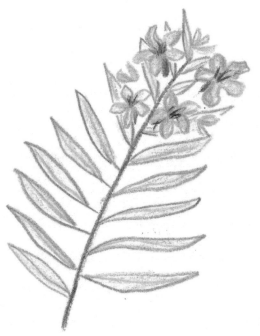

OLEANDER FLOWER

There are beautiful bushes all around our campsite with these bright pink flowers. I used my plant app to look them up (yes I have a plant app) and turns out it is called Oleander and is super poisonous.

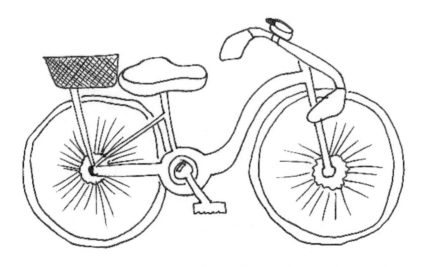

MELLOW VELO.

Today, we hired bikes and rode to the most western point of the island where there was an impressive lighthouse. The towns here are made up of beautiful white houses with colourful shutters and flowers growing up the side. It was the most stunning, tranquil ride and all three of us loved it, though Milo fell asleep on the way home and watching his little head bob up and down was hilarious. I could absolutely get used to this life.

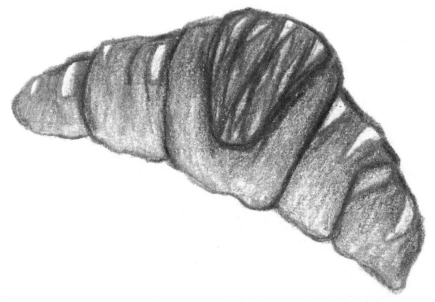

FRESH CROISSANTS.

This morning, Harry cycled into the town to get fresh croissants from the bakery. They were still warm when he arrived and we wasted no time tucking in. Milo eats his by holding each end and starting in the middle which makes me feel very uncomfortable, but hey ho, he's quiet! Not sure how he's going to cope when we get home and he doesn't eat them for breakfast every day.

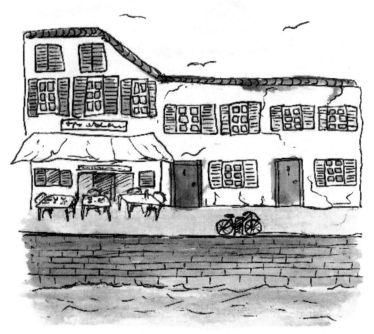

SAINT MARTIN.

Today, we cycled over to Saint Martin which was the most idyllic seaside town I've ever visited. Every street was like something off a postcard and the harbour was absolutely magical. I could have stayed forever.

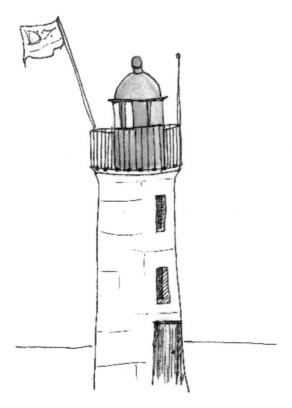

THE LIGHTHOUSE.

This morning, we had breakfast in the beautiful La Flotte looking at this lovely little lighthouse. We then headed back for a play in the pool before a final session at the beach and an incredible dinner at the beach bar with friends. I'm not sure how we're going to explain to this little beach babe that we have to go home....

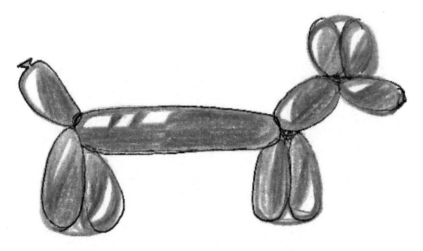

BALLOON ANIMALS.

Today, we set an alarm for 3:45am and crept out of our campsite with heavy hearts. We made our way to the ferry and arrived in time for check in. Milo found it all very exciting and we were delighted to find out that there was on board entertainment including a magician and live music, which he fell asleep through. Then it finished with a party on the heli deck. They were handing out balloons and Milo had to choose which shape he wanted. He went for a sword and was pleased as punch... for all of 3 seconds before deciding he actually wanted a dog. Cue me turning my hand to balloon magic and attempting to make a dog from the sword. The smile on his face was worth the trouble.... Then it popped, typical.

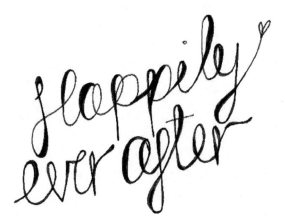

HOME.

Back home late last night which I thought would feel rubbish but actually was so nice. Waking up this morning in our own bed felt incredible. We then got to spend the day at the most awesome wedding of some lovely friends.

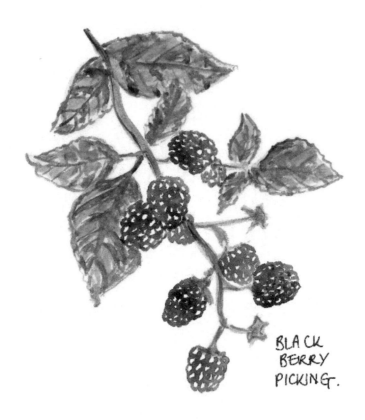

BLACK
BERRY
PICKING.

On our walk this afternoon, the blackberries were ripe and juicy and Milo enjoyed stuffing them into his mouth. I didn't mind as long as he kept walking, I wasn't far off leaving a trail behind me to keep him going.

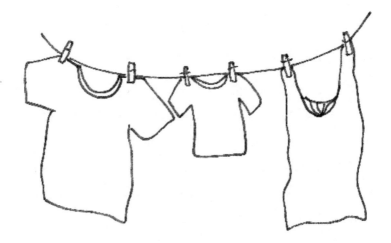

HANGING OUT THE WASHING.

Today, when I went back from my run, I was surprised to see that Harry had hung out a load of washing. I looked at him perplexed and he said he'd looked at the weather and it wasn't going to rain again. His optimism and positivity is what drew me to Harry when we met 12 years ago at uni. Mainly because I am the opposite, I prefer realist to pessimist but I guess they're the same. However, on this occasion I was right and while we were out, the heavens opened and gave our washing another good rinse.

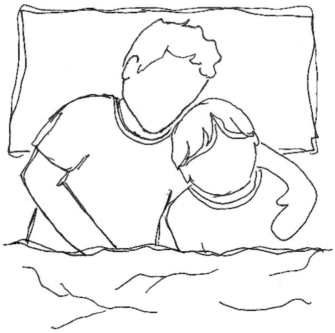

MUMMY CUDDLES.

Yesterday, Milo came home with a temperature and complaining of feeling cold. He'd been back at nursery ONE DAY. Poor little poppet was not well and was awake moaning and groaning most of last night. Unfortunately, he only wanted his Mummy so I spent the night cuddling up with him and trying to help him sleep. Though it was exhausting, there is nothing better than holding your bubba when they sleep, especially as they get bigger and it happens less and less often.

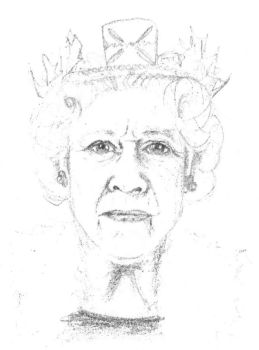

FOREVER OUR QUEEN

Whether you are a royalist or not, live in England or not, you will recognise what this woman did for her country. She was unfaltering for 70 years through wars and pandemics and showed what it means to keep calm and stay strong. Thank you for your service, Ma'am.

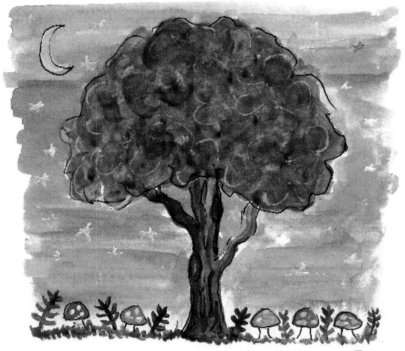

THE ENCHANTED WOOD.

Today was a busy day with the park, swimming and spending the afternoon with lovely friends. This evening I, feel absolutely shattered and when I put Milo down, I could have curled up with him to listen along with 'The Enchanted wood.' I'm not sure if it is the fact the he has dropped a nap, my Herceptin injection on Wednesday or the fatigue from chemo but I'm finding that by the end of the day, I.am.spent. Thank goodness for our comfy sofa and TV.

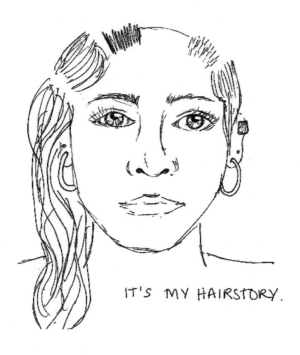

IT'S MY HAIRSTORY.

When I first met my oncologist, he said in a very casual, off hand way, "your hair will fall out. And then it will grow back." And to be fair, he wasn't wrong. It was a shock and I won't deny that it was hard at times, particularly when it started coming out in handfuls. It felt horrifying and made me feel like I was really sick. Being bald was actually pretty freeing and watching it grow back has been exciting. Recently, for the first time in a while, I actually look in the mirror and don't mind what I see looking back. I even decided to put on a bit of blond in because hey, why not?

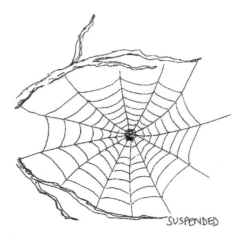

SUSPENDED

On our walk this morning, there was a layer of fog surrounding us and all over the gauze bushes were spiderwebs covered in water droplets. It was quite creepy and we crept closer to spot the tiny little spider perched in the middle of the web. I think spider webs are incredible and it amazes me how something so fragile can be so strong. At the moment, I feel suspended in a web of emotions, I flit between anger, elation, pure happiness, disbelief, gratefulness and fear. I feel suspended between the cancer world & the real world, between being healthy & sick and between the old me & the 'new' me. It's a strange space and as much I want to feel 'normal' again, it's taking me time to re-adjust. I know from speaking to others that this is all very common. Thankfully, I have found a great therapist to help me work through these things. Thank you to my wonderful friends and family for bearing with me.

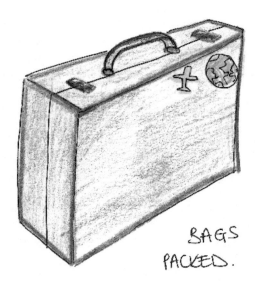

BAGS PACKED.

That's right, we're off on holiday again. Harry and I are going away to Sicily, just the two of us for the first time since our honeymoon 4 years ago. We booked it while I was on chemo to celebrate our anniversary, my birthday and, well, life. I'm terrified about leaving Milo for so long but he's in great hands and I think we need this. Also, a few people have asked me if I am going to keep this account going now that I'm recovering... when I set out on this creative journey, I set myself the challenge of doing one picture, everyday for a year, so my aim is to see it through. Thank you to those of you have joined me for this journey, I hope I have shed a little light and maybe made you laugh occasionally (rather than cry). Disclaimer: sadly, this is not what my suitcase actually looks like.

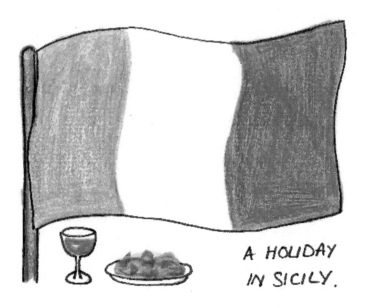

A HOLIDAY
IN SICILY.

After watching Stanley Tucci's 'Searching for Italy' earlier
this year and salivating the whole way through, we decided it
was about time we visited Italy and sampled some of the
incredible cuisine. We've come to Sicily after lots of
recommendations and are just about to pop out for our first
dinner. Also, if you haven't already, definitely watch 'Searching
for Italy' on iplayer, just make sure you've eaten first!

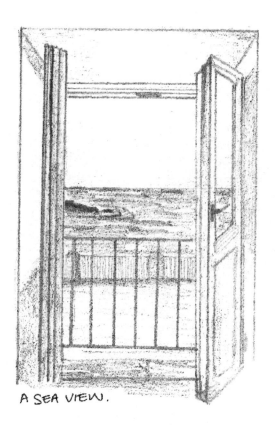

A SEA VIEW.

After a day lazing on the beach, we made our way down to
Siracusa and the Island of Ortiga to our beautiful hotel. It is
set in a stunning old building with high ceilings and stone floors.
The best thing is that our room has a view of the ocean and a
little balcony so we can hear the waves and watch people on
the street below. Feeling so, so grateful this evening.

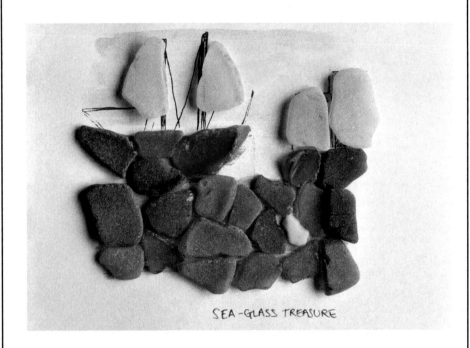

SEA-GLASS TREASURE

After spending the morning getting lost in the beautiful streets of Ortiga, we stopped for a delicious lunch and glass of rose. Then we spent the afternoon on the beach, most of which was in the shade, a relief from the heat, but some people were stretched out on the rocks like lizards basking in the sun. I was in treasure hunting heaven as the beach was covered in sea-glass. We caught the last of the sun at a bar in the square, bellissimo.

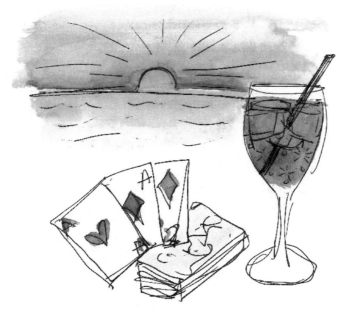

APEROL SPRITZ SUNSET

Today, we spent the morning exploring the archeological park in Siracusa before heading back to Ortiga for Calamari and Beers. Then, we cooled off in the sea and lay in the late afternoon sun before having a drink and watching the sunset. This evening, after another delicious dinner of pasta, we sat and watched some live music of covers of well-known songs (Wonderwall among them). Then on the way home, we stumbled upon an Italian band and though we had no idea what she was singing, we were drawn in and mesmerised. What a magical evening.

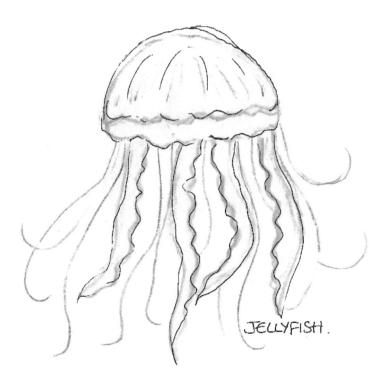

JELLYFISH.

This morning, we walked into the main town of Siracusa to the church where a Caravaggio painting of the death of Saint Lucia is displayed. After a lunch of giant, and delicious, arancini, we then spent the afternoon back on our favourite beach. While laying beached in the water to keep cool, I felt a little sting on my leg and looked down to see a little pink jellyfish floating away. Then couldn't get a song we used to sing at school with the kids out of my head.... "We are jellyfish, but we're not made of Jelly, and we don't look like fish, yeah"

(IYKYK)

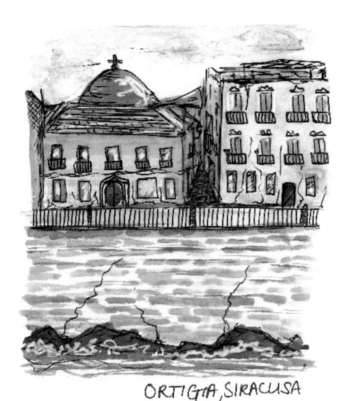

ORTIGIA, SIRACUSA

Today was my birthday and our last day so we got up (slightly) earlier for a swim. As I bobbed in the gentle morning waves, I looked back at the beautiful island of Ortiga. We spoiled ourselves with a delicious lunch of Caprese, antipasti and pistachio pasta. Then we spent our last afternoon with a final visit to the market and wandering the little streets before having an espresso in the Duomo. The perfect end to a wonderful holiday with amore mio!

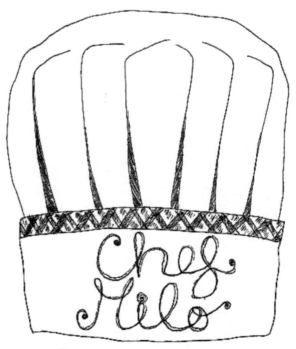

THE WAY TO MY HEART.

This morning, we set an alarm for the first time in a while and rushed over to my Mums to pick up Milo. He was so excited to see us and ran over for the biggest hug. It was just incredible to hold him after being away. We gave him his present, a personalised chef hat as he says he wants to be a 'food maker' when he grows up. I have always loved my food so take so much pleasure in watching him enjoy his. He loves to help out in the kitchen, even if he does sneak bits into his mouth and I love sharing a passion for eating with him.

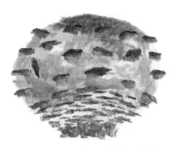

COMMON EARTHBALL

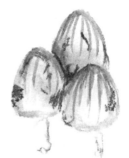

COMMON INKCAP

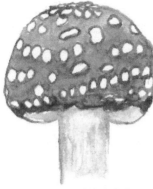

FLY AGARIC

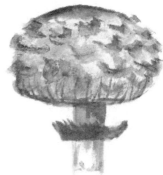

SHAGGY PARASOL

A BUNCH OF FUNGUS)

On our walks recently, we have been noticing all the mushrooms growing in the woodland around our house. I decided to find out what their names were and I was not disappointed.

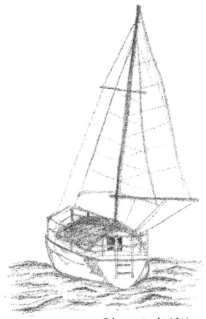

SAILING AWAY.

Today, my wonderful mother took me out for a birthday lunch. The restaurant was in a marina full of sailing boats and we sat in the gorgeous sunshine to eat our delicious food. I'm a lucky girl, thank you @braceyeileen . It's been just over 2 months since I had my 'all clear' and it feels like I am sailing away from a dark horizon, the further I get, the better I feel. I try to look forward and keep my eyes on where I am going but I find myself glancing back at the storm I am leaving behind.

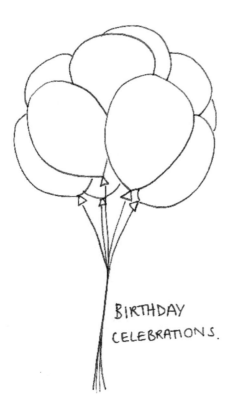

BIRTHDAY
CELEBRATIONS.

Today, I spent the morning dragging Milo around town looking for bits for his birthday party. It seemed impossible to find plain balloons but we got there eventually. This evening was spent eating delicious curry with some very special friends to celebrate the birthday of the group's elder.

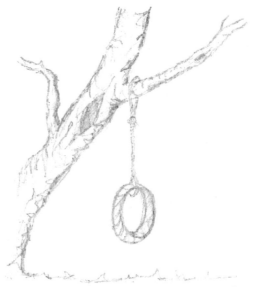

ROPE SWING.

Today was a day for cleaning our house, a task I have been putting off for about three months. (No judgement please). We then went for a walk on the common and stopped for a go on the rope swing. It's the perfect analogy for my mental health at the moment. I find myself constantly swinging between emotions - guilty and grateful, angry and calm, elated and devastated. It's absolutely exhausting (which is not helped by the insomnia - my fellow Tamoxifen takers know the pain of night sweats). Luckily, this evening, I am surrounded by my wonderful family and feeling loved.

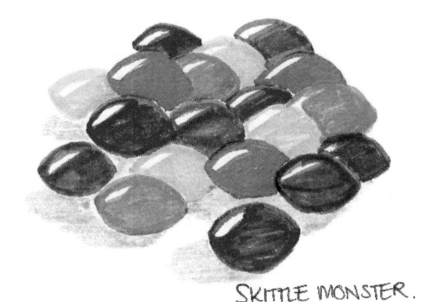

SKITTLE MONSTER.

Today, Harry's brother TJ and family arrived and Milo was so excited to see his cousins. We went for a walk and Milo was insisting on being carried so was grateful when TJ, who is a complete sweet-oholic, had a pocket full of skittles which he used to coax Milo along. Last minute preparations for the party this evening and now a Chinese and sofa!

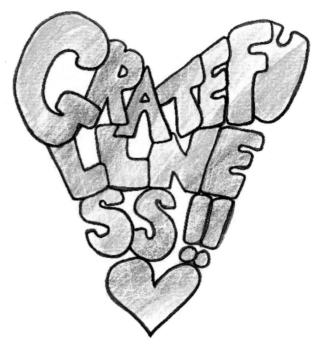

MY HEART IS FULL.

It's hard to describe how I feel after today but to say my heart is full seems the most appropriate. Surrounded by family and friends, we celebrated Milo's birthday with cake, a bouncy castle and balloons. He loved it and the look on his face was pure joy. This evening, after watching back the video of singing Happy Birthday, I choked. There were times during this year that I wondered if I would be around for special days like this, so grateful is an understatement. Thank you to all those that joined in the fun and helped out. Lovelovelove.

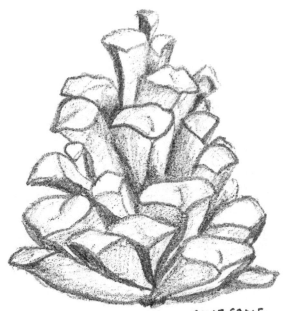

LUCKY PINECONE.

Today was my first day at uni for my Masters in Art Psychotherapy. Our first task was to go out and find an object to represent how we were feeling about starting this journey. I found a pine cone as we saw them all over in Sicily and found out that they were the local good luck charm. I felt it was good way to start this part of my life with luck on my side. It was wonderful to spend the day with a group of people who all feel the way I do about creativity and it got me so excited for what's the come.

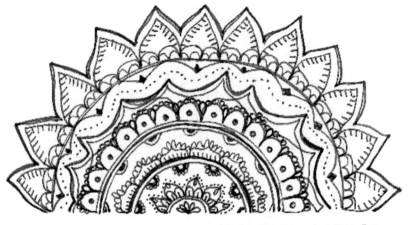

MULTIPLE LAYERS.

After another session with my therapist today, I have to come realise there are a lot of layers to my emotions and I have a lot to figure out. It's not until you start down the road of talking about how you view things and deal with problems that you realise how many defence mechanisms you have in place. I've always been a huge advocate for therapy and now that I am training to be one, it is part of the course that I attend weekly sessions myself for the next 3 years, so plenty of time to work through the layers.

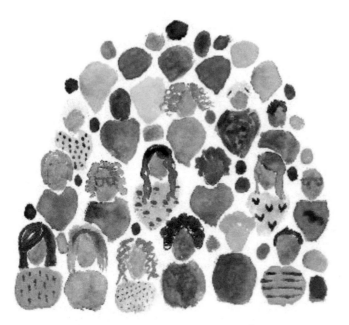

IT TAKES A VILLAGE.

While in hospital for my Herceptin jab today, I finally crossed paths with the lovely NikNakLou, who was diagnosed with stage 4 breast cancer, 5 years ago at the age of 30 and has been living life to the absolute full ever since(in between chemos that is). The people I have met on this journey have all been so wonderful and the support in this community is magical. It's like being part of an exclusive club and I feel so connected to people, most of whom I haven't even met in real life!

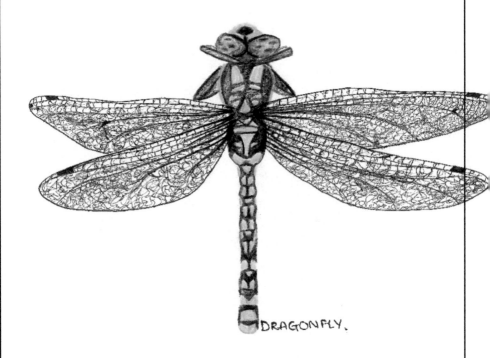

DRAGONFLY.

On our walk today, we spotted a dragonfly perched on a rock but when we got a closer look, we realised it was actually dead. I looked up what type it was and turns out it's a male 'Southern Hawker.' I don't feel like I've done the intricate, delicate wings justice but Milo was rushing me to join his game.

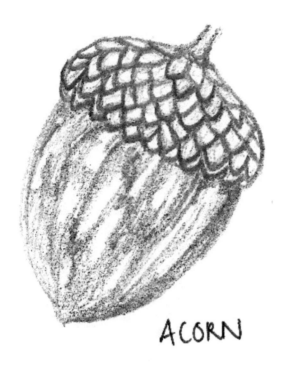

ACORN

Today would have been my Auntie Joan's birthday which makes me miss her terribly. However, one of my most favourite people welcomed a gorgeous baby girl into the world today and I am so unbelievably proud of her for being an absolute hero and can't wait to meet the baby girl. So this acorn seemed fitting today... it represents the end of summer as the leaves start to turn golden and brown. But it is also a new beginning, a new lease of life ready to start a magical journey in this crazy world.

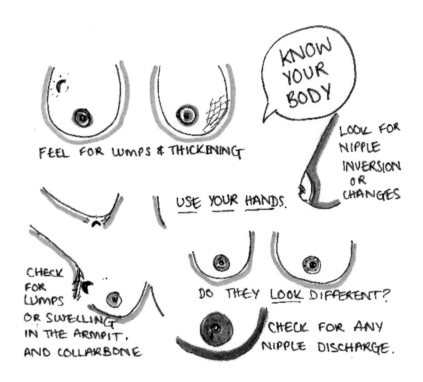

FEEL IT ON THE 1st.

Today marks the start of Breast Cancer awareness month so I thought I'd do a little doodle of the advice given on how to check your breasts. It's super important to know your body and be aware of any changes as picking up on something just might save your life. Not only this, with the NHS stretched more than ever, it can be hard to get your voice heard and taken seriously so if you know something isn't right, don't sit tight, don't 'see what happens' and don't keep quiet. Make sure you advocate for your health and your life.

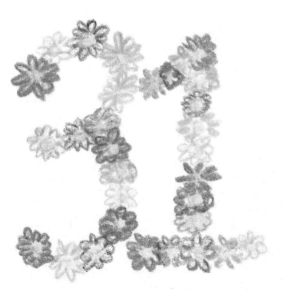

I STAND WITH THE 31.

31 flowers for the 31 women who die every day from secondary breast cancer in the UK. I stand by them and Met Up UK in raising awareness for secondary breast cancer. If you want to do/know more, please check out Breast Cancer Now Charity. Breast cancer is one of the most common cancer amongst women which is treatable, but at the moment, if it spreads through the lymph nodes to the rest of the body, it is known as metastatic, and it is not curable. I know some incredible women currently living with secondary breast cancer who are not only living life to the full but also campaigning tirelessly to #make2ndscount and to raise awareness and funding for more effective treatment.

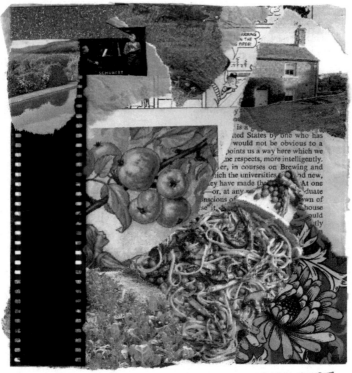

CULTURE.

Today, I travelled back up to London for my second day of uni
(I am on a part time course which allows me time for
placement, work, and looking after the little man.) We started
our first module in Placement Preparation and spent the
morning having an introduction to the theory behind Art
Psychotherapy. We were then asked to create a piece of art to
represent our 'culture' and I found myself drawn to the
natural world as well as food, literature, the arts and home.

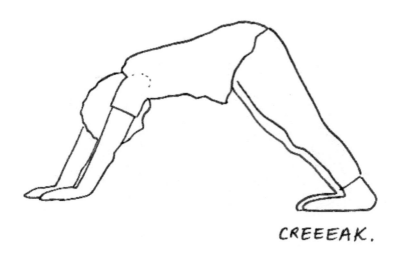

CREEEAK.

Tonight, I went to my first Pilates class in almost a year. I was looking forward to it as I feel like I've lost all my strength over the last few months. However, it was hard not to feel frustrated during the class with how little I can do in comparison to where I was this time last year. I know there is a reason for it but it was hard not to let the anger bubble up. Fortunately, by the end of the class, I felt calmer and I know that I just need to be patient with myself and channel the energy into regaining my strength.

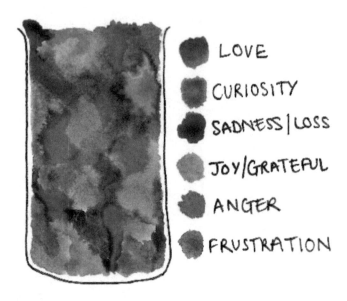

LOVE

CURIOSITY

SADNESS / LOSS

JOY / GRATEFUL

ANGER

FRUSTRATION

EMOTION - FULL.

My therapist remarked the other day that I clearly have a lot of emotions/feelings/thoughts buzzing round my head and that they spill out quite easily. This is how I picture that. Today I got to meet a very special baby and felt pure joy, but as I left, I felt sadness. They are so intertwined. Then on my run, when I struggled to get up a gentle hill, the frustration became overwhelming and I shouted "fucccck" before turning round to check I hadn't terrified a walker. It's a lot sometimes though I think this is the same for everyone and that it's about balance, finding space for all these emotions and being kind to yourself. On another note, if you haven't watched 'Inside Out,' you 100% should as it explains all this much better than me.

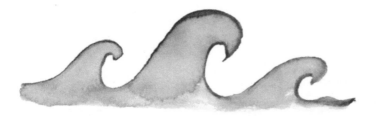

PART OF AN OCEAN.

Today, I took Milo swimming and at the end of our session they turned on the wave machine and as we bobbed along, I thought of the following story for the amazing book "Tuesdays with MORRIE"

The story is about a little wave, bobbing along in the ocean, having a grand old time. He's enjoying the wind and the fresh air — until he notices the other waves in front of him, crashing against the shore.

"My God, this is terrible," the wave says. "Look what's going to happen to me!"

Then along comes another wave. It sees the first wave, looking grim, and it says to him, "Why do you look so sad?"

The first wave says, "You don't understand! We're all going to crash! All of us waves are going to be nothing! Isn't it terrible?"

The second wave says, "No, you don't understand. You're not a wave, you're part of the ocean."

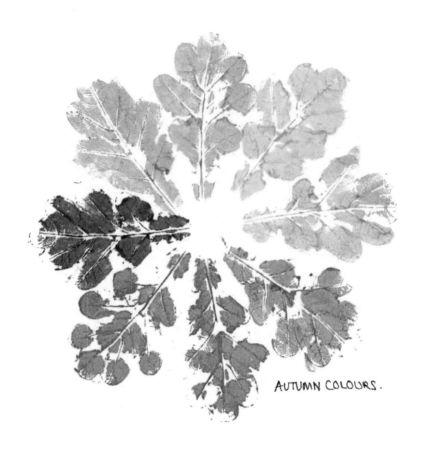

AUTUMN COLOURS.

It's that time of year again when the leaves turn the most glorious colours. On our walk today, Milo and I were crunching through the fallen leaves and acorns.

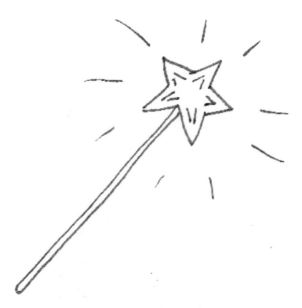

FAIRY GODMOTHER.

Yesterday, we went to the sweetest little farm with some lovely friends and their little ones. It was so fun and Milo loved feeding the Guinea pigs with my gorgeous god-daughter who, for my birthday, gifted me a 'Fairy Godmother' mug.

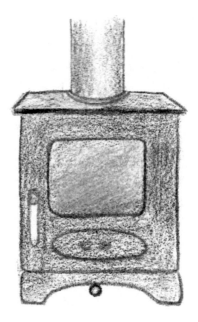

LOG BURNER.

Today was spent curled up the sofa after catching a horrible sick bug. It meant we had to cancel on friends who we were so excited to see but I had to give myself the time to rest and recover. Harry lit the log burner to keep me warm and as I lay there, it was hard not to feel like I was back in chemo days. I have to keep reminding myself that I will feel better tomorrow and that I am not actually back there. Thank god for Milo's cuddles and H looking after me.

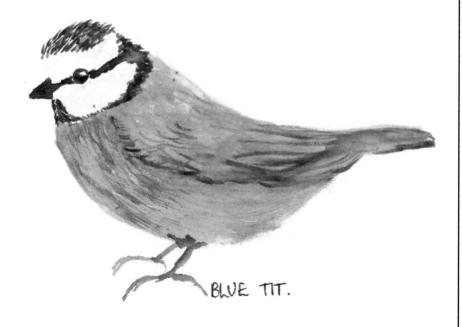

BLUE TIT.

I finally got round to putting some more seed out on the bird table and the birds showed their appreciation by hustling round it all day. The Blue Tits are the most common and are very cheeky in character. On another note, Harry said that this can be my new nickname for when I'm sad...

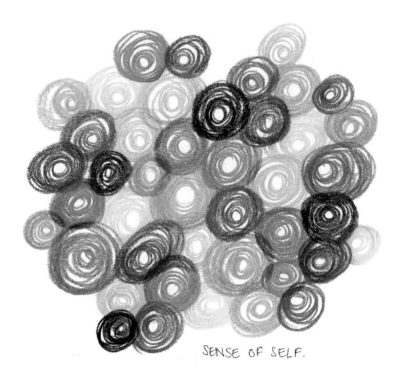

SENSE OF SELF.

Today, while doing my reading for this weeks lectures, I came across the following; "A person's sense of self arises from the experience of being on the mind of others....It is the intersection of the individual as they transect with others." It made me really think as I've always thought it to be important to have a sense of self based on my own value and told, "not to worry what others think." But it turns out, according to this text, that it is impossible to build a sense of self that is not somehow impacted by those around you. So pick your inner circle wisely.

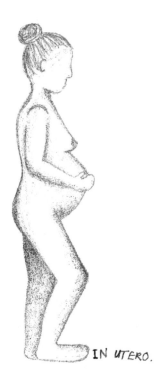

IN UTERO.

Today was an incredibly insightful day, learning about the human psyche and how research has shown that personalities can start to develop in utero and the attachment with the mother begins earlier than we think. It makes me think a lot about when I was pregnant and how I felt about my unborn baby. I also feel like a bit of foetus myself, in terms of my understanding of therapy and am looking forward to growing and developing over the next few years in my journey to becoming a therapist.

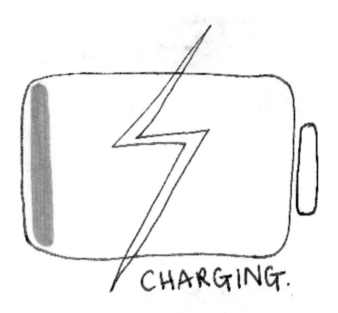

CHARGING.

After a full day of online lectures, it was so nice to get out for a walk with Milo and Moose this evening. Safe to say, I am completely and utterly exhausted. This is a word I have used a lot this year but tonight, it's a different kind. My body is tired but mostly my brain is tired. It's the kind of tired from listening, thinking and learning, which is so damn refreshing.

SUNSET SKIES.

The sky on the way home was so beautiful tonight and I found myself reflecting on the last few days at uni. Today was a heavy one, talking about mental health and trauma amongst other things. The final lecturer finished by reading a transcript from a session with a woman in hospital with terminal cancer. Listening to the way she spoke about, reliving all of those emotions and thoughts absolutely floored me. I felt like I was back there again and my body reacted in the same way; raised pulse, couldn't catch my breath, nausea. Luckily, I'm on the course with some incredible people and they made me feel so safe and supported, suppose that's what you get when you're surrounded by budding therapists!

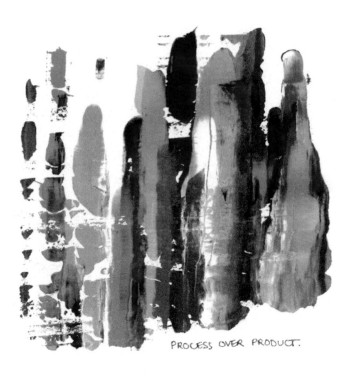

PROCESS OVER PRODUCT.

Now that I've had some time to think about my learning over the last few days, I have one, over arching thought. That when we focus on the product, we lose sight of the importance of the process. A little like the "it's the journey not the destination," we spend so much time these days thinking about our goals and what we want to achieve when it is the creative process itself which is the most rewarding. I can't say this really applies to the cancer journey, there is nothing particularly enjoyable about going through chemo and sometimes the end goal isn't as clear but it's what you can get from it that counts. Like the lovely Mikki said as part of her Asda campaign; "Grow through what you go through."

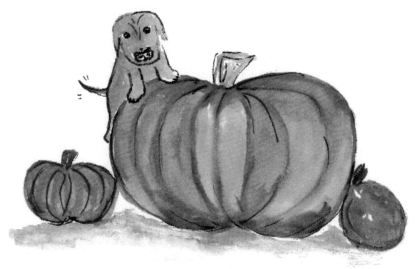

PUPPIES & PUMPKINS.

Today was a wholesome day spent with friends, petting puppies and picking pumpkins. Luckily, it was that way round as I'm not sure Moose would forgive us for bringing a puppy home, no matter how cute it was!

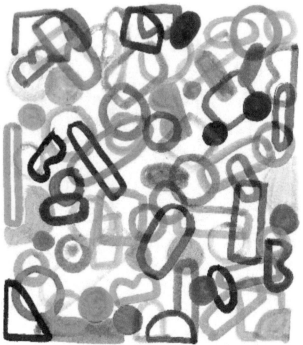

THOUGHTS & IDEAS.

Back up to London today, for another day at uni. I'm starting to get into the rhythm of it and loving getting to know the other people on my course. We are always sharing our thoughts and ideas and it's amazing to be surrounded by such caring and creative people.

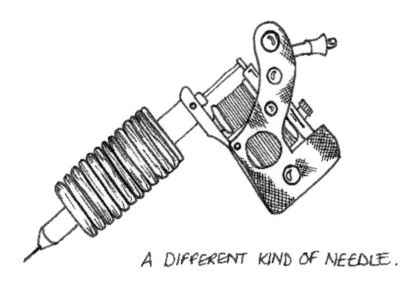

A DIFFERENT KIND OF NEEDLE.

So... I did a thing. After getting my Herceptin today, I headed over to Granny's Attic to have Kit do my first ever tattoo. It was incredible to take control and to mark my body with a symbol that meant something to me. It obviously hurt a little but it was my choice to be in that pain. The symbol is a line to represent the 'negative' result I received in July and the dot is a full stop to say that part of my life is finished. Also when I lift my arm, it becomes an exclamation mark as I plan to live life to the full from now on!

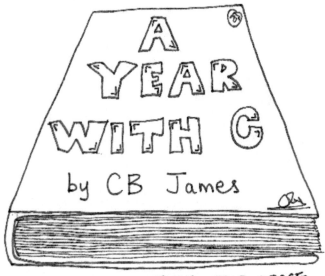

Coming Soon
to a Bookshop
Near you!

A YEAR WITH G
by CB James

WATCH THIS SPACE.

Today, I did something which excites me and terrifies me at the same time. I have found a publisher who is going to help me put these drawings & paintings together into a book. It feels like a good way to round off the year and I have spoken with them about setting up a donation to a chosen charity with every book. They have assured me that there will be something ready before Christmas for a pre order so watch this space!

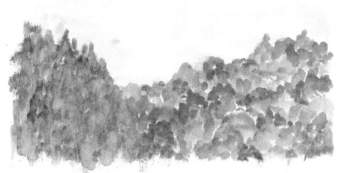

EVERGREEN & DECIDUOUS

On the drive back from a friends house this evening, I was in awe of the range of colours across the landscape ahead of me. I was having a conservation with Milo after he got frustrated that he couldn't open his snack bar properly (his frustrations usually revolve around food and not getting it into his mouth quick enough!) He persevered without my help, as I was driving, and managed to get it open himself. I congratulated him for not giving up and for persisting. Then I remembered one of our lectures at uni about resilience and how it is encouraged in order to cope with stressful times. However, our lecturer noted that rest is just as important as resilience. Rest is vital in order to recoup and process the increasingly pacy life that we all lead. There is a stigma around 'rest' that confuses it with giving up or being lazy. It is the complete opposite. Rest is as necessary as perseverance when it comes to survival in this mad world.

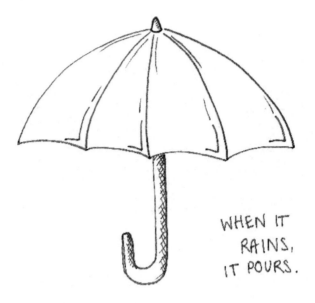

WHEN IT
RAINS,
IT POURS.

God almighty, the rain was ridiculous today. It felt like every time I stepped outside, it absolutely tipped it down. This phrase is often used when bad things happen in your life in quick succession but actually it's fitting for positive things too. After spending the first half of this year sitting round and 'resting', now I feel like all these amazing things are happening, all at once. It feels a little overwhelming this evening but I know that I just need to break it down into bite size chunks.

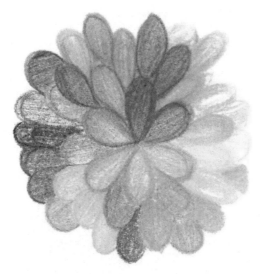

COLOUR WHEEL.

After a busy day of walks, lunch and gardening, I feel spent this evening. Doesn't help that I've caught Milo's cold. In other news, to celebrate my cancer-versary (a year from diagnosis for those that haven't heard this charming word before), my Mum and I have decided to walk a half marathon from her house to a pub near mine, to raise money for Breast Cancer Now.

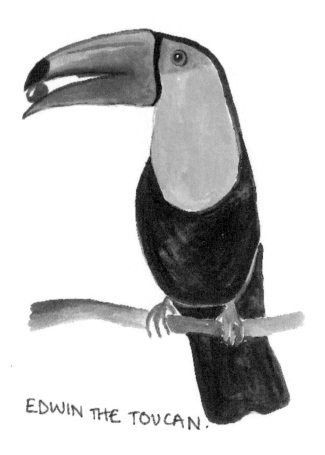

EDWIN THE TOUCAN.

Today, we met up with my brother & gorgeous fam and went to The Living Rainforest. It was a magical place and we saw a sleepy sloth, cheeky monkeys and a Green iguana (that was actually orange?!) but my favourite was Edwin the Toucan who was skilfully catching blueberries and grapes in his mouth.

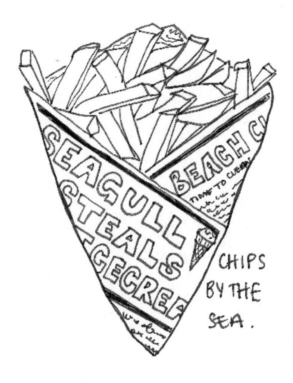

CHIPS BY THE SEA.

Today, I took Milo down to the beach to meet up with a wonderful friend and her son. The boys played on the pebbles, picking up shells and running in and out of the waves with Moose. Milo and I sat on the wall to share our chips while the seagulls circled above us. It was one of those days that was so simple yet so special and my heart felt full. There is something about having your life dangled which makes you slow down and you enjoy being in the moment.

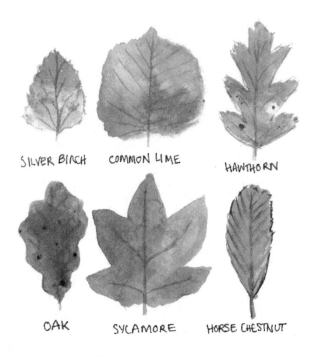

SILVER BIRCH   COMMON LIME   HAWTHORN

OAK   SYCAMORE   HORSE CHESTNUT

TYPES OF TREES.

On my walk today, I couldn't take my eyes off the carpet of fallen leaves, admiring the beautiful range of colours. I realised I could only identify the oak leaves, so when I got home, I dug out our leaf guide from the Woodland Trust. Fun facts; Silver Birch sap can be used to make wine and beer, oak was used to make the ships in the Battle of Trafalgar and Horse chestnut is named so because it was supposedly used as a horse medicine.

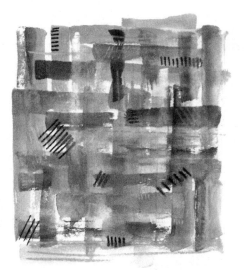

ABSTRACT.

I've been chatting with a lovely fellow breastie, Talia, recently about how we have both ended up doing something completely different after cancer. She used the term "Post Traumatic Growth" which describes positive psychological change that comes after a stressful life event. I prefer it to "the silver lining" which seems far too pretty and simplistic when paired with cancer. Though, saying that I am very grateful that despite the shitstorm that is cancer, it has led me to start my dream career.

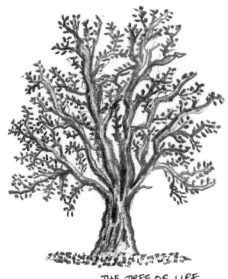

THE TREE OF LIFE.

Last week, Mum took me to a talk about a local artist, Adrien Hill, who was a war artist, focusing a lot of his work on the destroyed trees on the battlefield. Later in life, he contracted TB and ended up in hospital for a long period. During his convalescence, he would paint and draw in order to pass the time and found it to be extremely therapeutic. Hill then encouraged the other patients on the ward to do the same and found that it helped them too. This was the start of Art Therapy in the UK and he is known as the founder. In Hill's later years, his love of trees brought him to my neck of the woods (see what I did there) as there are some incredibly old Oaks around here. The Queen Elizabeth Oak Tree is thought to be 800-1000 years old. Astounding.

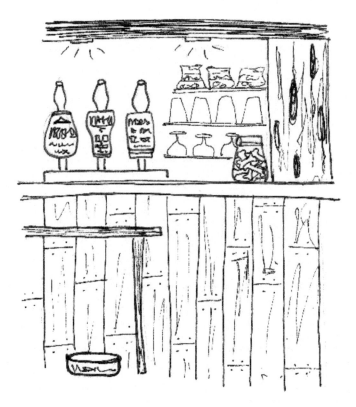

THE PUB.

Today, my dearest friend and Milo's godmother arrived for a visit. We took the dogs out for a walk up on Blackdown then headed home to make pizza for tea. Harry messaged on his way home from work suggesting a drink at the pub, so we popped to our local for a pint. Ya can't beat it.

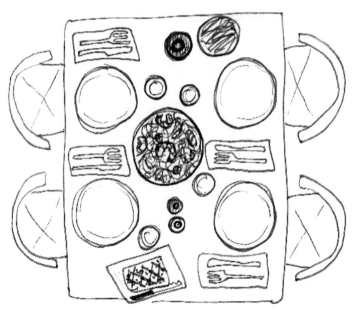

DINNER WITH FRIENDS.

Today, after a lovely morning helping some dear friends move into their new house, we headed up to London to see some very special friends. Milo loved it as we got closer and could spot the red buses and cranes looming above us. We arrived and Milo was so excited to see two of his (and ours) favourite people. After a Halloween themed treasure hunt and dance party, Milo was bathed and bedded so we could sit down for the most delicious dinner. There really is nothing better than catching up with wonderful friends and eating incredible food.

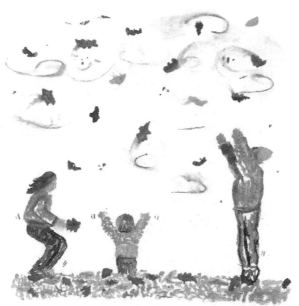

CATCHING FALLING LEAVES.

Today, Rory and Ish took us to Beckenham Place Park which was absolutely gorgeous. We wandered through the Farmer's Market before heading into the park where we played the game of trying to catch a falling leaf, as it supposedly brings good luck. Turns out it is much more difficult than you think and it's all about waiting for the big gusts of wind then running round in circles like headless chickens. It was bladdy hilarious and we were proud that we all managed to catch one (except little Milo, bless him). Sometimes it feels like life is a swirling, whirling chaos, but you just gotta embrace it, reach out and grab a leaf.

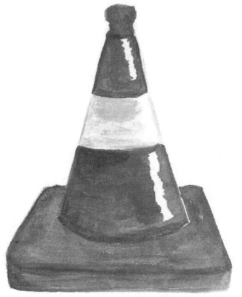

DIVERSION.

On my way up to uni today, I got stuck in traffic. For about 20 mins we crawled along, only to discover that the cause of the delay was that one of the lanes was blocked by a line of cones. I actually laughed out loud at how ridiculously annoying it was but something my Mama once said popped into my head. "There will be lots of debris when you are floating down the river, you just have to learn to move around it." Happy Halloween!

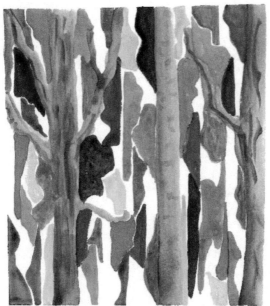

THE LIGHT BETWEEN THE TREES.

Well, November started with a bang, didn't it?! We had torrential rain, hail, wind and thunder and lightning. Moose and I managed to find a break in the weather to go out for a walk in the woods.

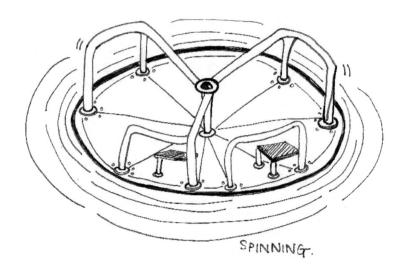

SPINNING.

Today was my first day on placement at a local Special Needs school. It was the most incredible place and the children were so sweet. One boy in particular, just wanted to spend all of playtime on the roundabout. It was pretty hard to push but the look of sheer joy on his face made it absolutely worth it, even it did make me dizzy! After spending most of this year not having to think about much, I am finding that my head is spinning with all the different things I've got going on. All good things but it can feel overwhelming at times. Thank goodness for chocolate.

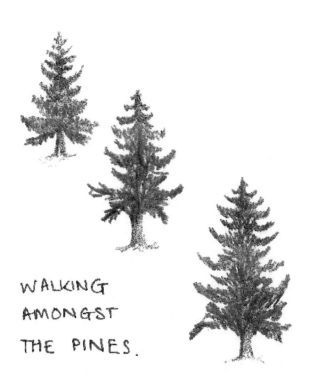

WALKING
AMONGST
THE PINES.

We took advantage of the sunshine this afternoon and went
for a long walk up in the pine woods. On the way back down,
the sun was setting and the clouds were lying low in the fields.
It was a mystical.

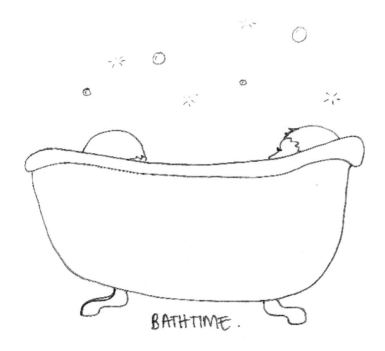

BATHTIME.

At the end of most days, Milo and I have a bath together and debrief the day. Mainly, I go over what we spent the day doing and ask him questions to which he replies "nothing!" then finds himself hilarious. Tonight, I am exhausted and couldn't say much and instead just watched him play. Harry arrived home and I started to cry. I am absolutely drained at the moment. I feel like I have gone from 0 to 100 recently and though there are so many exciting things happening, I am struggling to keep all the balls in the air. Luckily, I saw some of my favourite people today so will hold that in my mind and get an early night.

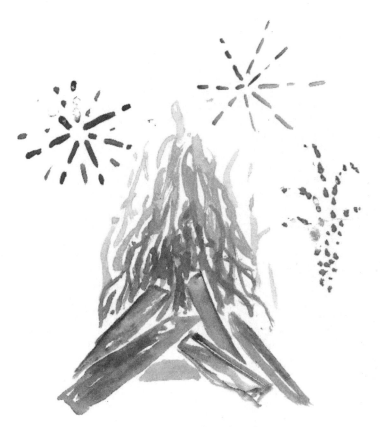

BONFIRE NIGHT.

We're down in Somerset this weekend with some of the most wonderful people in the world. They say that when it comes to the people in your life, you have radiators and drains. Tonight, I am surrounded by warmth.

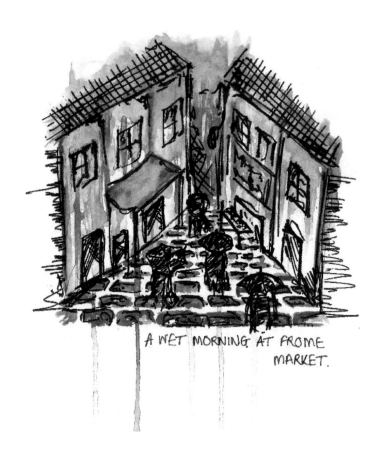

A WET MORNING AT FROME MARKET.

We spent the morning exploring Frome Market, admiring all the talented local creatives. Unfortunately, the rain was relentless and we got soaked to the bone within minutes. Luckily, after sheltering in the pub for some lunch, the sun came out and we were able to peruse the stalls with more ease. I ended up falling in love with a print by the amazing artist David Daniel.

DRIP, DRIP, DRIP.

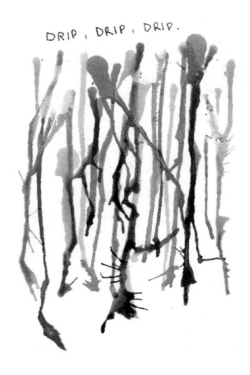

More rain today. Luckily, I could watch it from the warmth of my studio where I spent the day as uni was online. Today, we were talking about how babies develop and the importance of the relationship with the primary caregiver. It's hard not to reflect back and think about Milo and how he coped this year.

As a parent, you are constantly thinking about your child/children, a little like a dripping tap. So going through cancer as a parent was unbearable at times and I often worry about the impact on him. However, we also learned today the importance of the other caregivers in a child's life, which made me smile to think about the wonderful people who took over and swept Milo up when I wasn't able.

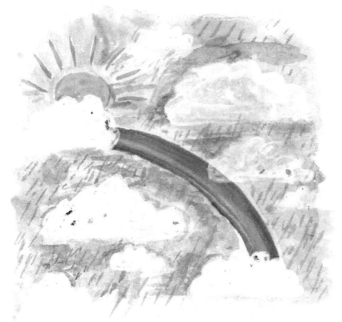

RAIN BEFORE RAINBOWS, CLOUDS BEFORE SUN.

Tonight, at bedtime, I read Milo one of his favourite stories that my Mum bought. It really helped me over the last year and still brings tears to my eyes whenever I read it.

Rain before Rainbows,
Clouds before sun.
A day full of promise, a day full of light,
The morning is breaking and the morning is bright"
- Smriti Halls and David Litchfield.

SCAN-XIETY.

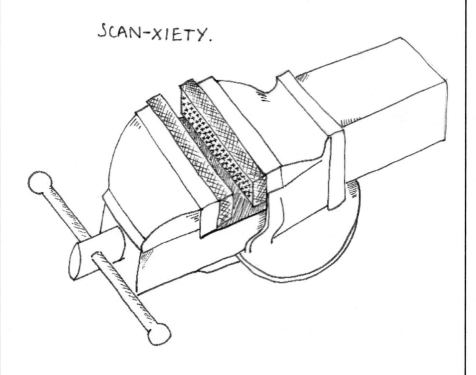

Today, I was back in the hospital for my injection and a mammogram. I have to have one to check my remaining breast, at least once a year, unless I notice anything strange. I know that it is a good thing and that I'm lucky they want to check but the experience is awful. Those that have had a mammogram will know, the machine is a monster vice which your breast is roughly placed into then tightened by the technician. You then have to stand there awkwardly, clamped by your boob while they take an X-ray photo before finally being released. A form of torture. I had put it out of my mind but then saw

it on my calendar for today and the anxiety started. The last time I was in one of these machines, it was for 45 mins (lying down) while they took 12 biopsies of my breast. Not only that, but when you see bad results on a scan, you can't help but expect those every time. I managed to suppress my anxiety, but it started tightening this morning then when I walked into the room, it hit me and I physically shuddered at the sight. Luckily, I only have one breast to scan so it didn't take long and the technicians were friendly. Now it's the agonising two week wait for the results but at least no more clamp for another year.

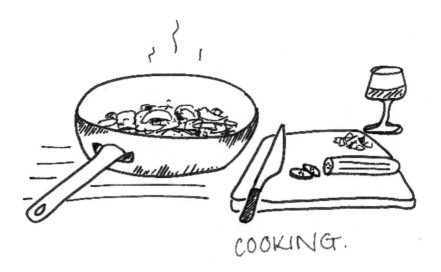

COOKING.

After a busy (but lovely) day, Harry arrived home slightly earlier than usual meaning he could take Milo up for bathtime and I could cook dinner. Some days, I can't imagine anything worse than putting food together to form an edible meal. But tonight, it was cathartic to chop and slice while I enjoyed a glass of wine in peace.

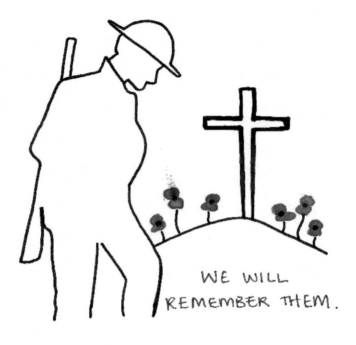

WE WILL
REMEMBER THEM.

We drove up to visit my brother and fam this morning so Milo could have a play with his cousins. Rather aptly, my brother is in the army so it seems appropriate to spend Remembrance with him.

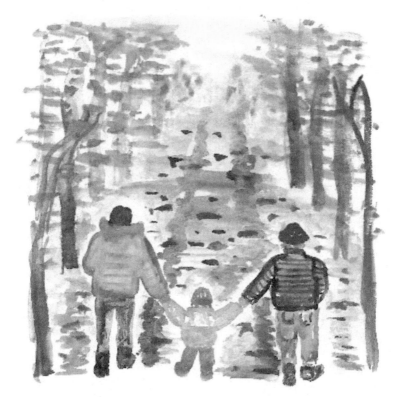

AUTUMN WALKS AS A FAMILY.

This afternoon, we walked to one of our local pubs in the gorgeous Autumn sunshine. Once there, we met some of our favourite people and chatted over cheesy chips. Perfection.

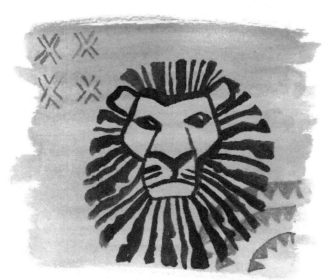

THE LION KING.

Today was a very, very special day. We travelled up to London on the train then the tube (Milo couldn't quite believe his luck) to meet Harry's family. We started with lunch at the Jungle Cave which the kids loved. Then we headed to the theatre to see the Lion King. I was a little nervous that Milo was going to get bored/scared but he was amazing. Watching the joy on his face as the animals walked passed us down the aisle to the 'Circle of Life' brought a tear to my eye. His Aunty Tara bought him and his cousins a little baby Simba which they all lifted up when Rafiki did on stage, absolutely adorable. I've always loved the theatre myself so seeing him enjoy it so much was amazing. Thank you Grandma and Poppops for such a wonderful Christmas present and memories that I will cherish forever.

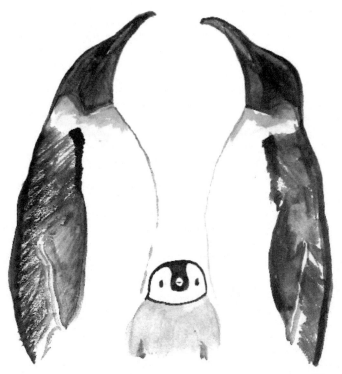

THE EMPEROR PENGUIN.

Last night, we watched Frozen Planet II which was incredible as expected. I particularly enjoyed the bit with the Emperor Penguins who live in the harshest place on earth and yet prioritise family above anything else. They go on an unbelievable journey in order to find a mate, protect an egg and then chick from the strongest, coldest winds in the world. The hardship they endure is unimaginable yet they persevere.

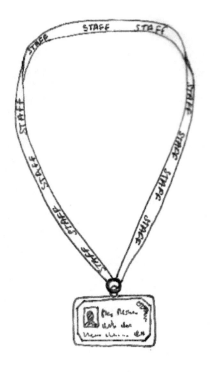

IDENTITY.

Today was my first day back at work since I was diagnosed almost a year ago. It was only for the afternoon but I was so nervous and apprehensive as the last time I was there, I got the phone call saying I needed to come in to the hospital right away. However, when I arrived today, I was greeted with such gorgeous smiles and kind words that I instantly felt fine. It was so good to get back another bit of myself.

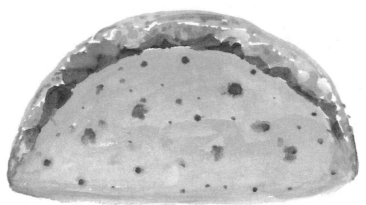

TACO WEDNESDAY.

There are days when my mind goes blank on what to draw.
Today was one of those days. Too tired to think, so I painted
the Tacos I cooked for dinner. Happy Hump Day everyone.

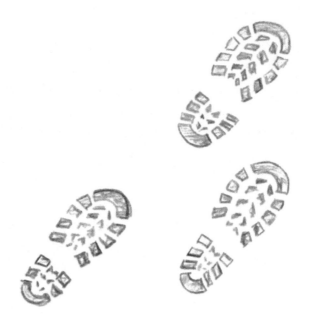

MUDDY FOOTPRINTS.

So much mud. The ground is so slushy from all the rain and today, I made a total tit of myself by driving our 2-tonne van onto grass and instantly got it stuck. Doh! Luckily, a friend was nearby with his truck and came to my rescue. My brain is like mud at the moment. Struggling to hold on to thoughts and make sensible decisions (like NOT driving off road). Sleep it is then.

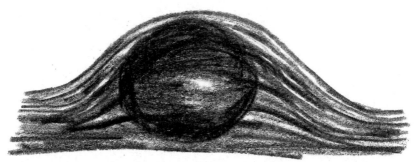

A LUMP IN THE ROAD.

On this day, one year ago, I drove to the hospital for an appointment with a breast consultant to check my lump. I'd already gone up, 2 weeks before, but the Dr was running more than an hour behind and I had to leave to get Milo. So, second time around, I walked into the Drs office and she did her examination. She looked concerned and sent me down to have an ultrasound. Off I went down the long corridors and my anxiety was beginning to rumble. I'd been feeling off for a few weeks and had horrible acne on my chin. I knew my hormones were off kilter. After a short wait in Radiotherapy, they called my name. As I lay there on the bed and stared up at the ceiling, I had a heavy, dark sensation building in the pit of my stomach. The radiographer squeezed on the gel then rolled over the lump. As soon as I saw it on the screen I knew it was bad, but the look on her face confirmed my fears. This did not look good. She then proceeded to check my lymph nodes and found one to be enlarged... another concerned look to her technician. She then explained she would take some biopsies and that I needed a mammogram.

A few jabs with what sounds like a staple gun then I was hustled into the X-ray room for the boob clamp. I was ready to burst into tears but held it together, it felt completely surreal. Once they were finished, I left the hospital and burst into tears on the phone to my mum. She tried to persuade me not to imagine the worst, but I knew deep down what was coming. I rang Harry and he tried to do the same, cover it in sunshine and rainbows but I lashed out and said that I just needed his comfort and to be told that it was going to be OK.
To look back and think what has happened since then is madness and in the course of my life, is hopefully going to be a blip that I can grow from. As Lizzo said, "Speed bumps only make you aware" They most certainly do.

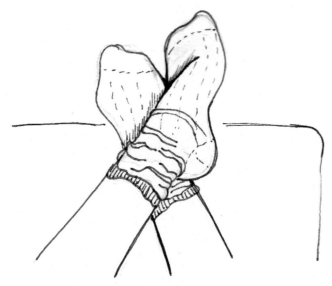

FEET UP.

After a very busy but heart-full kind of day, I have the house to myself this evening as Harry is out at the rugby. It's a rare treat to be able to sit quietly and reflect in peace.

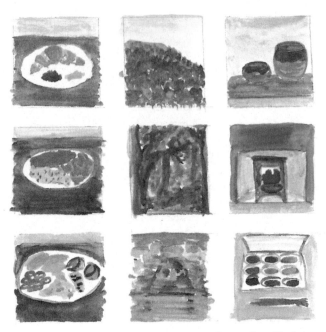

SUNDAY FUNDAY.

What a busy day of walks, delicious food, craft fair and wonderful friends. Mum and I did a section of our walk for next weekend and the views were beautiful.

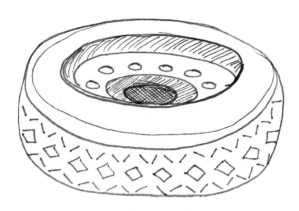

SPARE TYRE.

After an exhausting day at uni doing lots of thinking about thinking, I was ready to get home, have a cup of tea and a cuddle with Milo. Unfortunately, the universe had other plans and 5 mins from home, there was a loud bang and my tyre popped. I pulled over and got out in the wind and rain to begin changing it to the spare. Despite my best efforts, and mincing my hand, I couldn't loosen the bolt and had to call a friend who was nearby to come to my rescue. Not the way I wanted to end my day but luckily my mum and brother are here this eve so good company and delicious food. (Adding to my spare tyre!)

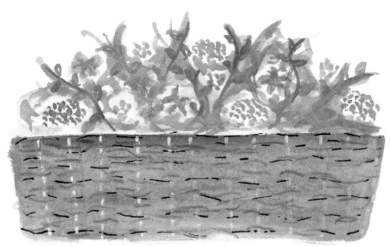

THE MOST BEAUTIFUL GOODBYE.

Today was Harry's Grandma Michele's funeral. She was a beautiful, kind and graceful person which was reflected in a service full of song and light to celebrate her life. The church was packed and everyone had stories to tell about her kindness and joy for life. It's a little reminder that life is not about how successful you are but instead how many lives you touch and the light you bring to others.

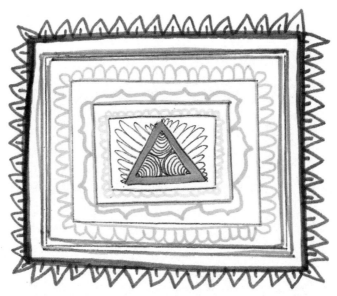

THE THERAPEUTIC FRAME.

This afternoon, while Milo was at nursery, I had some time to have a crack on my first essay in almost 10 years.... We have to write about our understanding of the "Therapeutic Frame" which is part of the foundations of Art Psychotherapy. The concept is that the triangular relationship in the middle between therapist, client and art is contained within a well bound frame in order to make sure that the therapy is safe and facilitating. We have learned a lot about boundaries and how to make them clear and defined. This is something I am trying to practice in my own life, being able to put my own boundaries in place. And occasionally say "no."

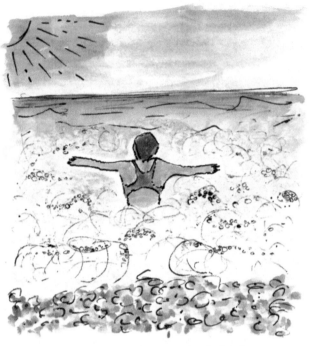

SEAS THE DAY.

Today marks a year since I was diagnosed with Breast Cancer. On that horrible day, I was at school when I checked my phone at lunch to see a missed call and a voicemail. When I listened to it, my heart froze. It was a consultant at the hospital asking me to come in that afternoon to see her. I knew that didn't mean she had good news for me. All my fears had been confirmed and I rang my mum to let her know and ask her to have Milo then Harry to tell him to meet me there. The optimism in him tried to reassure me and again I told him clearly, to expect the worst. Sure enough, when we arrived, the doctor's sombre face said it all but when she finally said the word "cancer," the gasp from Harry will live in my memory forever. I gripped his hand as she explained that we did not yet have all the information but that it was fast growing and things were going to move quickly from now. I tried to take in as much as I could but I had gone numb.

I didn't cry there and then, just bit my lip and toldmyself I could do this. A year on, after 7 rounds of chemo, many many different drugs, 3 hospital stays and a mastectomy, I am a different person. Today, I went for a dip in the stormy sea and faced it head on. Quite symbolically, I got knocked down by the force of the wave but I had a smile on my face - I knew I could get back up. I have been given a second chance to live my life to the full and I shall be forever grateful.

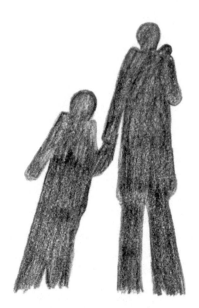

MY LITTLE SHADOW.

One of my first thoughts when I was diagnosed was Milo. Despite telling myself regularly that there was no way I was going to let it happen, I wondered about him growing up without me. Though it was one of the hardest bits about going through treatment, worrying about the impact on him and not being able to be the mum I wanted to be, having him by my side gave me strength. Even on the days when I was dizzy with exhaustion and nausea, he was there to make me smile and keep me going. I'm not in any way saying that it was easy for him, some days I was so awful and snapped at him unnecessarily but we are stronger than ever and I have so much appreciation for the little moments we have had together, like our walk in the sunshine today. It's a shame he won't be with me for the whole walk tomorrow but he'll join for the last stretch and of course, the celebration drink in the pub!

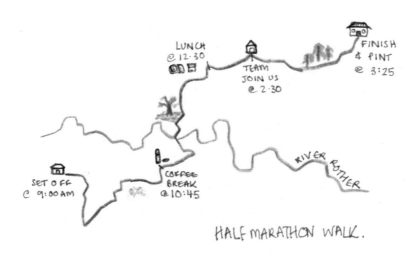

LUNCH
@ 12.30

TEAM
JOIN US
@ 2.30

FINISH
& PINT
@ 3:25

SET OFF
@ 9:00 AM

COFFEE
BREAK
@10:45

RIVER ROTHER

HALF MARATHON WALK.

Wow, what a day. So so thankful for all those who joined us, supported us and celebrated with us. It was such a joyous day and I almost burst into tears at the end. What a journey. I am overwhelmed with the love that had been sent my way today and over the last year. I will never be able to eloquently put into words how much it means to me, but I will be forever grateful.

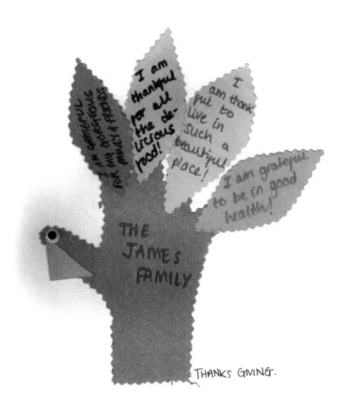

THANKS GIVING.

Today we got invited to our first ever Thanksgiving and spent the afternoon with friends, old and new, chatting and eating delicious food (first time having sweet potato with marshmallows). Before we sat down, the friend who was hosting us got us doing some crafts with the kids, she's a primary school teacher like me, we love an organised art activity! We had to make a Thanksgiving Turkey and after the weekend we've had, it wasn't difficult to think of things that I am grateful for.

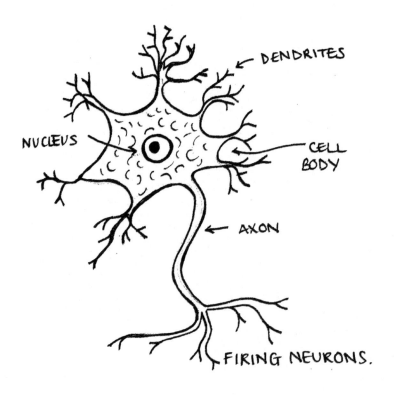

Today's learning was about the brain and how the environment we grow up in has a profound effect on the way the brain develops. I find it fascinating. Neurons fire all the time for a huge variety of things and form the pathways so that we can think and feel and do. I read in the text book that a piece of brain the size of a grain of sand contains 100,000 neurons. Mind blowing. There is so much about the brain that we still don't fully know or understand but one thing I know for sure is that mine in frazzled.

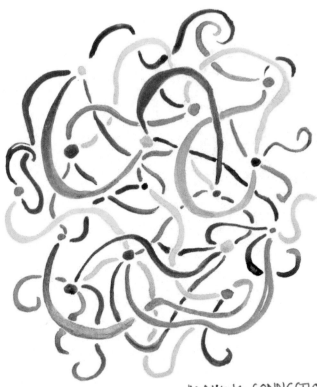

MAKING CONNECTIONS.

Yesterday, I got the opportunity to take part in some collaborative art. It was an amazing experience as we sat on the floor and mark made it silence, occasionally checking it was okay to encroach on others space. We'd been having a discussion about children's tv shows before so the colours certainly reflect that but I loved how we all took on similar themes. I have met some really wonderful people on this course and even though I only see them once a week, I am getting to know them better and better each time. A wonderful bonus to this course. In other news, got the results from my recent scan today.... No signs of cancer in my left breast! Wahoo!!

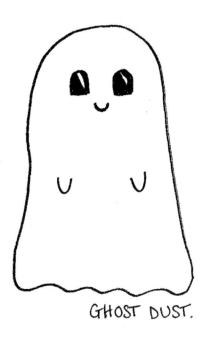

GHOST DUST.

On our drive home, the fog lay thick on the road in front of us. Milo remarked, "look at all that fog mummy, where did it come from?" To which I explained that it is like low lying clouds and he replied, "no! I think it's Ghost Dust." I think this is a much better word for fog personally. Also, a good description for my brain these days, after getting a message from my chemo nurse while at school earlier, asking if I was still planning on coming to the hospital for my injection. I had completely forgotten. Felt so useless and frustrated with my inability to hold information in my foggy brain. Damn that chemo ghost dust.

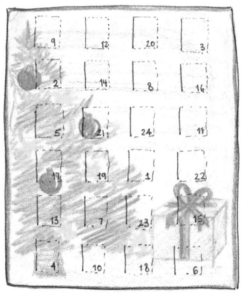

ADVENT CALENDER.

After a busy day of soft play and swimming, my mum popped
round this afternoon to drop off an advent calendar for Milo.
Where on earth did December come from?!? Feel like I've been
putting off thinking about Christmas and suddenly we're on
the count down. Milo couldn't believe his luck when he found
number one (turns out he recognises some numbers now, proud
mama) and tucked into the chocolate. However, I've had to
put it up high as I caught him trying to open another one
while I was making dinner. Little monkey.

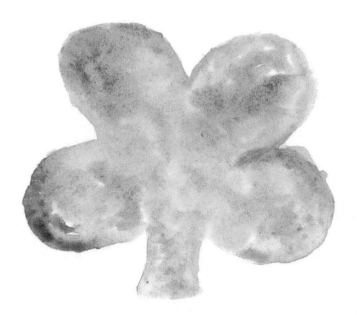

LUCKY BUT UNLUCKY.

After a play at the park this afternoon, we were walking to the van when I heard a hissing sound. I looked down at the tyre of the van and realised it was going flat. FFS, really?! REALLY?! Another flat tyre?! How unlucky am I?!? It's funny, a few people have said to me recently that I am 'lucky but unlucky' and I totally agree. Despite it being a rather crap year, what I have been given is priceless. I have had waaaay more time with Milo than I ever would have got if I'd been working. I've had so many walks in the woods like the one this morning, with my two favourite little ones and for that, I feel lucky.

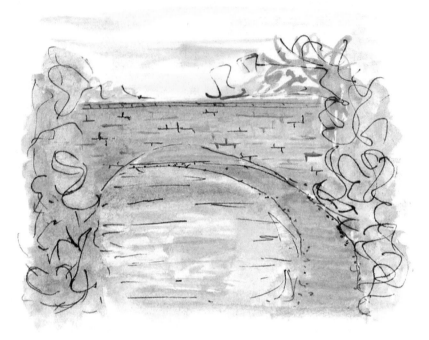

A WALK ALONG THE CANAL.

This weekend, we are up with Harry's family in Warwickshire and this afternoon we all went for a lovely walk along the canal. One of the amazing things about meeting someone is gaining another family.

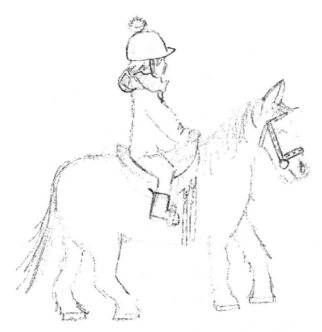

CLIP CLOP CLIP CLOP.

Today, Milo had his first ever horsey ride. He's been asking to for ages and the last time he tried, he was too scared. This time, he gripped tightly to the saddle while the pony plodded along and he quickly got used to the bumpy ride. I was so proud of him for being brave and felt emotional as I watched him clip clop along the road. Feels like my little baby is growing up so fast.

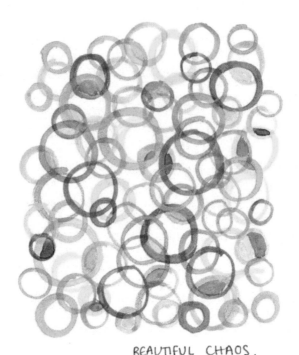

BEAUTIFUL CHAOS.

At uni today, we were in a group session and discussing how we were all feeling. The general consensus was "overwhelmed" - with our first essay due next week and most people still struggling to find placement, on top of the sound of sleigh bells as Christmas fast approaches, we were all feeling a lack of control. We then spent the afternoon watching a documentary film called 'In Utero' about all the things that can influence us in early life and it just reminded me that life is absolute chaos.

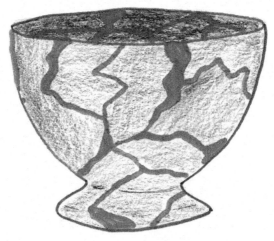

BROKEN.

The other day, I read something about how a disco ball is made up of broken glass (mirrors) and used to spread joy (and awesome dance moves). It made me think of Kintsugi, the Japanese art of repairing broken pottery with gold. It reminds us that our scars and broken parts are not only part of who we are but bloody beautiful.

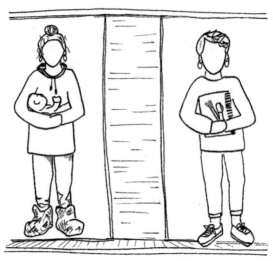

SLIDING DOORS.

If you haven't seen the film "Sliding Doors," I recommend it. The premise is a woman who either catches or misses a train and that split second thing changes the course of her life. We get to see both eventualities play out and how that tiny moment completely changed the direction her life went in. I've thought about it a lot this year as often I think about what I would be doing if it weren't for the cancer. We had planned to start trying for another baby at the start of this year, so I imagine that I would have had the baby by now (had everything gone "to plan") and be in that dreamy but crazy phase of shuffling around the house in pyjamas and a top knot, stuck in a feeding, changing and sleeping cycle. But instead, I am becoming an art therapist and publishing a book. Neither is better nor worse, just different paths, and I am grateful to be on this one.

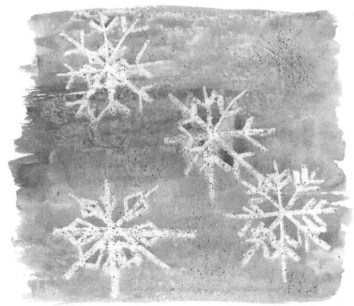

THE FIRST FROST.

Brrrrr, it's getting cold out there! This morning was the first time this year I had to hurl a saucepan of warm water at the windscreen to melt the frosty ice. Milo loved it and couldn't take his eyes of the intricate icicles on the windows. Each of them is completely unique which is breath-taking. I created this piece using oil pastels and watercolour over the top, children tend to like the method as it's like 'spy' writing.

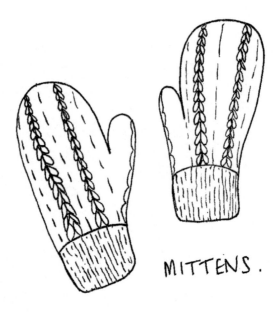

MITTENS.

This evening, we went to the magical Wisley Glow. Despite half the group missing to illness and the rest of us going in an hour later than planned due to horrendous traffic, it was amazing. I was worried about me and Milo getting cold so we put about 30 layers each and even dug out our matching mittens. We visited this time last year with my family and went for a pub lunch before, then Harry and I had to race to the hospital to meet the oncologist for my treatment appointment before re-joining the group to head into the gardens. It was surreal and I remember walking round trying to distract myself from the year ahead with the pretty, twinkly lights. This year, I had no treatment plan in the back of my mind and enjoyed making all the appropriate "oooo" and "ahhhh" sounds with some of my favourite people.

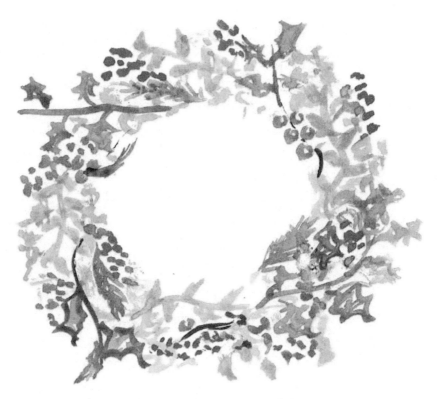

CHRISTMAS WREATH.

Christmas has officially arrived in our house, the tree is up,
Christmas ratty is out and this afternoon, Mum came over so
we could make our wreath together while sipping on mulled
wine. Cosy and content.

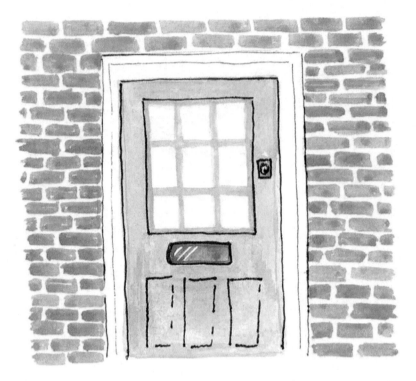

A NEW FRONT DOOR.

This morning, bright and early the guys arrived to fit our new door. It wasn't ideal with the temperature outside at -2 but it was amazing of them to come out on a Sunday. Not only do we absolutely love it but it is SO much warmer than the old one which is extremely helpful in this ridiculously cold weather we are having.

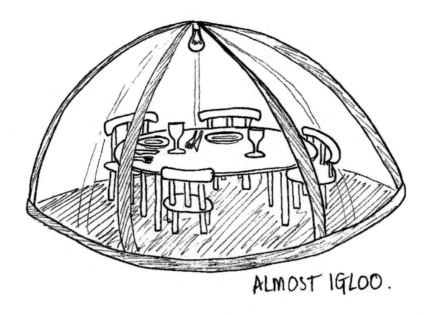

ALMOST IGLOO.

Tonight, I went to meet a friend at the Coppa club for dinner. We first met over 3 years ago now while we were pregnant and have been close ever since. We had planned to sit outside in one of their igloos this evening, but the cold was too much to bear, so we changed plans and came inside. She's also had a curve ball thrown at her this year and watching her deal with the challenges with so much strength and dignity, while still being able to have a laugh is awe inspiring.

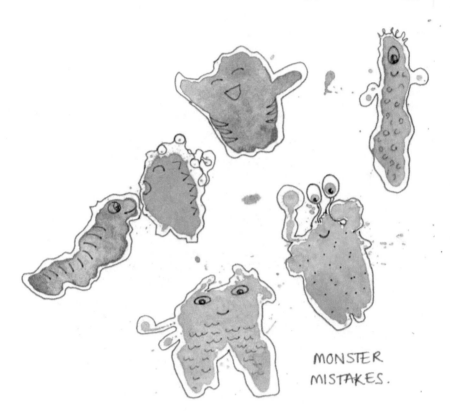

MONSTER
MISTAKES.

While writing (and rewriting) my essay today, a line stuck out to me; "there is no such thing as a mistake in art therapy and that everything that happens has significance and meaning." I think this is applicable to all mistakes in life and they are not to be ashamed of but instead are something to learn from. These little monsters were so fun do, super easy too, just splotch some paint then doodle away.

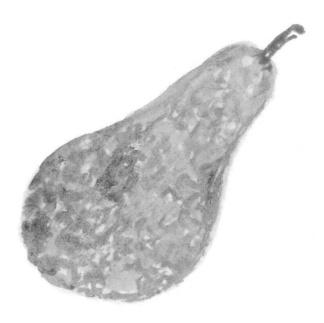

WHAT A PEAR.

On Monday, I had an appointment with my consultant to check my scar and discuss my scan results. After doing an examination, she said that I was healing well and couldn't feel any signs of reoccurrence which is good news. She asked about reconstruction and I said that at the moment I had no interest in putting my body through another surgery. I've got used to only having one breast and it doesn't bother me as much as I thought it would. I know this may sound strange to some, but it is my new normal and I want to get on with my life, even if it is pearless.

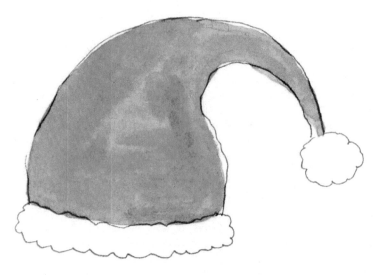

THE REAL FC.

Today, I took Milo to his nursery as Father Christmas was visiting. We sang Christmas songs, then when he arrived, the children excitedly waited for their name to be called. He was wearing Nike trainers and his beard had broken so he was holding it up, but the kids didn't seem to notice and were swept up in the magic of it all. Oh, to be so young and innocent. This evening, I'm seeing some of my most favourite girls for delicious food and wine.

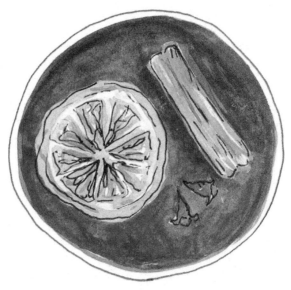

MULLED WINE.

After a busy day of shopping and a 1st birthday party, we've travelled up to the in-laws for the weekend. I've completely lost my voice which is no surprise so this evening when I was offered a drink, I went for a warm Mulled wine to soothe my throat. It's my absolute favourite drink this time of year and I can actually smell today's painting! A hearty meal of sausage, mash, and gravy and I am ready for bed.

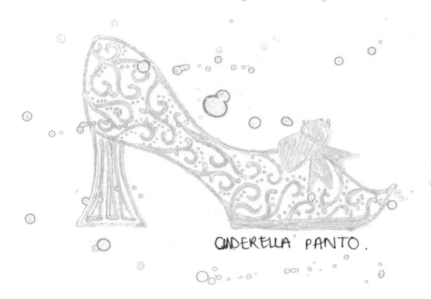

CINDERELLA PANTO.

Today, we went to the Cinderella Pantomime with the James fam and it was absolutely hilarious. Milo lapped it all up and we enjoyed the adult humour. After a delicious meal in Pizza Express, we are all together this evening drinking bubbles (hence why I spelt Cinderella wrong). Though, I've always been terrible at spelling... I mean, if the shoe fits...!

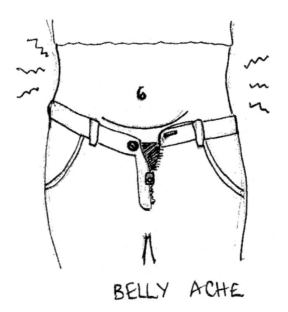

BELLY ACHE

I'm not sure whether it was the ab workout this morning, the ridiculously large and tasty Christmas Meal or the fact I spent all weekend laughing with the James clan, but this evening my belly aches so much so that I've had to undo the button on my jeans. Full belly and full heart.

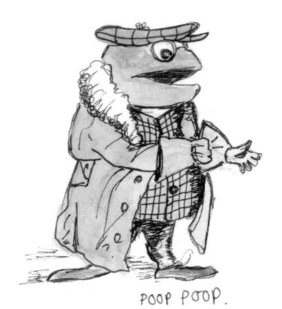

POOP POOP.

Another day and another amazing show and this time it was 'Wind in the Willows' with Milo and Nana. Despite not feeling very well, Milo sat beautifully for most of it and enjoyed the costumes and songs. The favourite character was obviously Mr Toad who had us all in stitches. Milo LOVES his catch phrase, "Poop Poop." More memories to cherish.

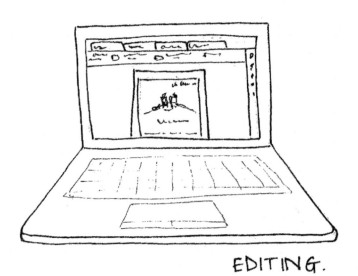

EDITING.

For the last few weeks, I have spent evenings sat in front of my laptop, scrolling through the book manuscript and making small editing notes. I was starting to lose sight of why I was doing it when I received the foreword, written by someone very special to me. It reminded me not only why I love this person so dearly, but also the reason I am putting my illustrations and words together to form a book.

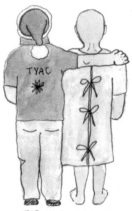

THE REAL HEROES.

Today, in between Christmas shopping, I popped into the hospital to get my injection. As I walked through the chemo ward, admiring all the twinkling lights and Christmas decorations, I noted it was as busy as usual and had a realisation. Cancer (and all other illnesses in fact) does not care about Christmas, so the staff were carrying on as usual while wearing their Santa hats and tinsel. I arrived at the TYAC ward and the nurses were all there having lunch together, celebrating the head nurse Claire's last day. She was the one who set up the Teens and Young Adults Cancer ward all those years ago and has been at the hospital for over 20 years. She came out to chat with me about her travel plans and asking about me, while I waited for my jab. She then ended up doing it herself as the other nurse Sam had to tend to another patient. The strength and kindness of nurses is phenomenal and I am in awe of what they do, day after day, despite the impact it must have on them. Though, I'm sure others will agree, the staff of TYAC really are one in a million and total superstars.

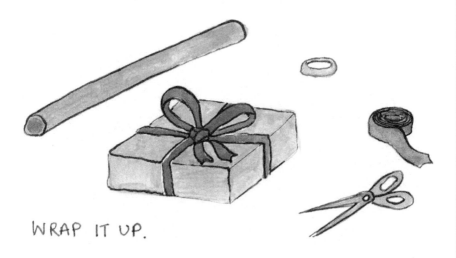

WRAP IT UP.

Last night, while Harry helped me to wrap all the Christmas presents, we talked about how many days left I have of this project. When I decided to start it, almost a year ago, I wasn't sure if a) I was going to be able to keep it up and b) if anyone would be interested in joining me on this creative journey. I've been blown away by the messages I have received from total strangers this year, which along with support from family and friends have encouraged me to keep the project going despite having doubts about its impact. Now that I am on the countdown to wrapping it all up, I am pleased I persevered and proud of what I have accomplished. Hopefully, come January, I can tie it all up in a bow in the form of a book.

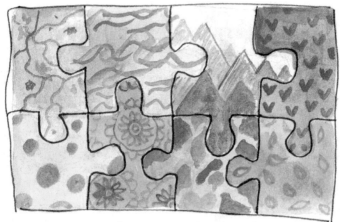

LIKE A JIGSAW.

Today, we have travelled to Wales to have Christmas with my family. Whenever we get together, it is total chaos; a mix of arguments over games, too much food and drink, nutty children & dogs and walks in the rain. I'm sure most families are the same, but we have all grown up to be unique individuals yet somehow fit together again (for a short while) like a jigsaw. On that note, I'm off to start our traditional Christmas jigsaw puzzle.

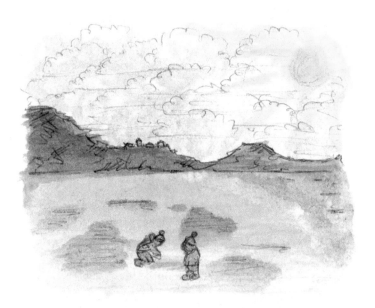

CHRISTMAS EVE BEACH WALK.

Today, we took a walk along Llangenith beach with cold winds and winter sun. The boys played in the puddles and we listened to the crashing waves. (Didn't fancy a dip this time!) Then this evening, we all sat down to watch Charlie Mackesy's 'The boy, the mole, the fox and the horse,' and I tried not to cry throughout. What an amazing work of art, brought to life so beautifully. My favourite quote from it is "One of our greatest freedoms is how we react to things." It couldn't be more true, in my opinion. This evening the children got into their Christmas pyjamas and then set up the tray of treats for Santa and co. Now, he's a little older and knows what is going on, it is so nice to see Milo enjoying the magic of it all.

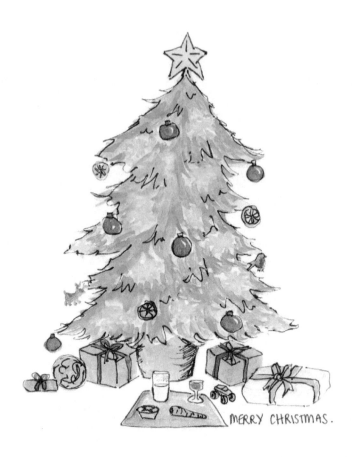

MERRY CHRISTMAS.

Merry Christmas, everyone! I hope you have had a lovely day
surrounded by friends and/or family. After spending a day
helping the little ones open their presents (the favourite was
a plastic monstrosity disguised as a Monster truck track,
which the boys barely left alone all day), and eating a
ridiculously good Xmas dinner, we've finally sat down in front of
the fire to open our secret Santa presents.

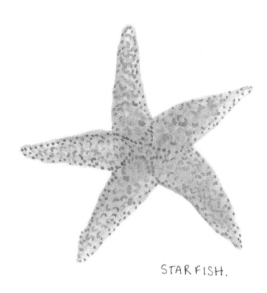

STARFISH.

Today, we drove over to my favourite beach in the world, Three Cliffs Bay. The sun came out as we arrived so we ate our turkey sandwiches, played in the sand and stacked stones. Then we wandered over to the arch and on our way through, spotted a gorgeous little starfish floating in a rock pool. The boys stopped to stare in wonder as it gave us a little wave. Days like today will never be forgotten, absolute magic.

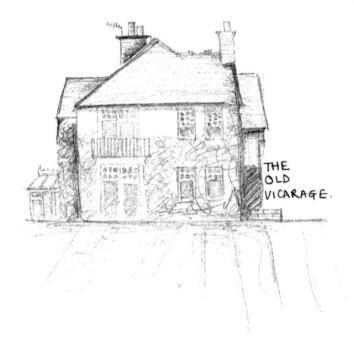

THE
OLD
VICARAGE.

Today was a rainy day so we spent most of it inside, enjoying
our amazing holiday rental house that my mum found. It's a
very old property with creaky floorboards, open fires and
beautiful high ceilings. Harry and I attempted a run in the
sideways rain and we were rewarded with a trip to the local
pub with views of the sea.

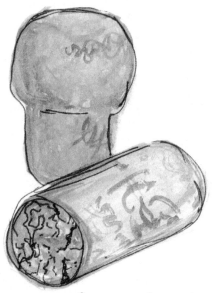

BOUCHON.

Today, my cousins arrived with their boys and the house is a bustle of love and good energy. Harry and I cooked a curry this evening which went down well and now we are setting up to play card game 'Bouchon' (French for cork) which involves collecting 4 of a kind then grabbing a cork from the table, of which there is one less than the number of players. (Also known as 'Spoons'). Let the hilarity and mayhem commence.

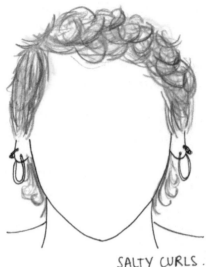

SALTY CURLS.

Today, I took my last swim of the year at the beautiful Oxwich Bay. I ran down the beach with the encouraging shouts from Milo and the rest of my family. As I dived into the icy water and my body shuddered in shock, I was reminded again what it has been through this year. 7 rounds of chemo, over 40 injections into my tummy & 10 into my leg so far, 6 months of hormone therapy and lymph node surgery + single mastectomy. Despite the fact I occasionally look in the mirror and don't recognise/like what I see, on the whole I am unbelievably proud and impressed with my body and what it has withstood. When I was diagnosed with cancer, I felt a disconnect with my body and a sense of "why are you trying to kill me?!" And it has taken a long time to move past that feeling. As I struggled to catch my breath and the waves towered above me, I felt no fear at all. Just a sense of relief that at last I feel in control. For the rest of the day, my hair was set by the salt and the short curls were blowing in the wind.

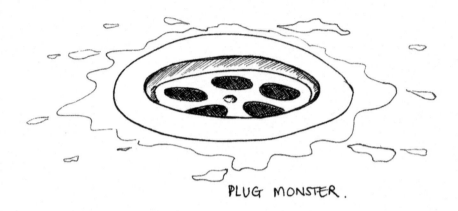

PLUG MONSTER.

Today, we bid farewell to my family and our beautiful Welsh house, then set off for home. The journey along the M4 was slow and boring but arriving home was worth it. After a flurry of unpacking, lighting the fire and building piles of washing, we all jumped into the bath to warm up. It was a squeeze, but Milo loved it, especially when the overflow tap started gurgling. We always get him to "awaken the plug monster" to drain the bath which he loves but you can tell he is slightly scared of the gurgling sounds, but it gets him out of the bath quicker!

The plug monster in my head is awakened whenever I feel a twinge in my shoulder, a bump in my armpit or notice a spot on my chin. I immediately start thinking that it is happening all over again. I can feel myself sinking into the fear of reoccurrence and I have to grab hold of something to ground myself. I'm sure as each day passes, this will happen less and less. Though I am going to be super careful and check my body often, I refuse to live my life looking over my shoulder (or in my armpit in fact!) Life is simply too short.

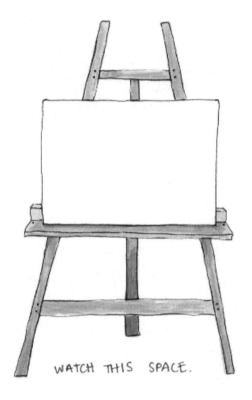

WATCH THIS SPACE.

This year has been one of the best and worst of my life. I have had times when I have been at my absolute lowest and thought I wouldn't be able to celebrate Christmas with my family or be sat here, bringing in the New Year with some of my favourite friends. However, there were also times this year where I have never been happier and have created memories that I will cherish forever.

This creative journal has been a challenge but on the whole has been amazing and I have enjoyed sharing my journey with all of you. Though at times, I felt narcissistic and that I was fishing for sympathy, I was reminded time and time again by friends, family and people I have never met that it has had a positive impact in some way. It has been such a big part of my year and helped me in more ways than I can count. It gave me a sense of purpose and direction when I felt completely lost.

A million thank yous to all the wonderful people in my life who have got me through this year with a smile on my face including my incredible families, caring friends and amazing health care team. I will be eternally grateful for all of you.

So what will I choose to fill my 2023 canvas with...
I could run every day,
or do yoga,
or learn a new skill...
The possibilities are endless but whatever I do, it is my choice and I choose to live.
Every. Single. Day.

Printed in Great Britain
by Amazon